Wissenschaftsethik und Technikfolgenbeurteilung
Band 13

Schriftenreihe der Europäischen Akademie zur Erforschung
von Folgen wissenschaftlich-technischer Entwicklungen
Bad Neuenahr-Ahrweiler GmbH
herausgegeben von Carl Friedrich Gethmann

T0224106

F. Breyer · H. Kliemt · F. Thiele (Eds)

Rationing in Medicine

Ethical, Legal and Practical Aspects

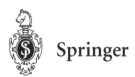 Springer

Reihenherausgeber

Professor Dr. Carl Friedrich Gethmann
Europäische Akademie GmbH
Wilhelmstraße 56, 53474 Bad Neuenahr-Ahrweiler, Germany

Bandherausgeber

Professor Dr. Friedrich Breyer
Fakultät für Wirtschaftswissenschaften/Statistik
Universität Konstanz, 78457 Konstanz, Germany

Professor Dr. Hartmut Kliemt
Fach Philosophie, Universität GH Duisburg
Lotharstraße 63, 47048 Duisburg, Germany

Dr. Felix Thiele
Europäische Akademie GmbH
Wilhelmstraße 56, 53474 Bad Neuenahr-Ahrweiler, Germany

Redaktion

Friederike Wütscher
Europäische Akademie GmbH
Wilhelmstraße 56, 53474 Bad Neuenahr-Ahrweiler, Germany

ISBN 978-3-642-07670-1

Die Deutsche Bibliothek – CIP-Einheitsaufnahme
Rationing in medicine : ethical, legal and practical aspects / eds.: Friedrich Breyer ... .
Berlin ; Heidelberg ; New York ; Barcelona ; Hongkong ; London ; Mailand ; Paris ; Tokio : Springer, 2002
  (Wissenschaftsethik und Technikfolgenbeurteilung ; Bd. 13)

Springer-Verlag Berlin Heidelberg New York
a member of BertelsmannSpringer Science+Business Media GmbH

http://www.springer.de

© Springer-Verlag Berlin Heidelberg 2010
Printed in Germany

Coverlayout: de'blik, Berlin

Printed on acid-free paper   62/3020Hu - 5 4 3 2 1 0 -

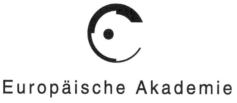

Europäische Akademie

zur Erforschung von Folgen wissenschaftlich-technischer Entwicklungen
Bad Neuenahr-Ahrweiler GmbH

The Europäische Akademie

The *Europäische Akademie GmbH* is concerned with the scientific study of consequences of scientific and technological advance for the individual and social life and for the natural environment. The Europäische Akademie intends to contribute to a rational way of society of dealing with the consequences of scientific and technological developments. This aim is mainly realised in the development of recommendations for options to act, from the point of view of long-term societal acceptance. The work of the Europäische Akademie mostly takes place in temporary interdisciplinary project groups, whose members are recognised scientists from European universities. Overarching issues, e.g. from the fields of Technology Assessment or Ethics of Science, are dealt with by the staff of the Europäische Akademie.

The Series

The series "Wissenschaftsethik und Technikfolgebeurteilung" (Ethics of Science and Technology Assessment) serves to publish the results of the work of the Europäische Akademie. It is published by the Academy's director. Besides the final results of the project groups the series includes volumes on general questions of ethics of science and technology assessment as well as other monographic studies.

Foreword

The book series on the ethics of science and technology assessment edited by the Europäische Akademie is devoted to the publication of the work-reports of its project groups, works on the foundations of ethics, the philosophy science, and other issues related to the work of the Europäische Akademie. In addition, the series comprises the proceedings of conferences organized by the academy.

The 13th volume documents the proceeding of the academy's spring symposium in 2000 on Rationing in Medicine which was held in Bad Neuenahr-Ahrweiler on March 23–25, 2000. An intense discussion on the future of health care in Europe has been stimulated by increasing difficulties of securing adequate and needs-orientated medical care in the face of scarce resources and medical progress. Unfortunately, quite often a rational discussion of rationing is drowned out by the political talk of the day. But only an open and well-informed debate, if anything at all, can lead to transparent and just rationing procedures which eventually might be acceptable to the public at large.

For this debate much can be learnt from observing the experiences other countries have made with their health care arrangements. What kinds of mistakes should be avoided and what might be useful in the different states and perhaps also in the supra-national context of an emerging Europe are interesting and important issues.

Where is rationing heading? Though nobody can know precisely, we are in need of bold conjectures drawing scenarios of effective and nevertheless acceptable rationing schemes. The academy's conference aimed at stimulating the debate on rationing in medicine by interconnecting German experiences with the international context. We hope that this volume – bringing together papers written by scientists from fields like medicine, law, economics and philosophy – will contribute to the understanding of the present state and future development of rationing in medicine.

Bad Neuenahr-Ahrweiler, July 2001   Carl Friedrich Gethmann

List of Authors

Baurmann, Michael, Professor Dr. phil., studied sociology, philosophy and law at the Johann-Wolfgang-Goethe-Universität in Frankfurt. 1983 doctoral thesis on Rationality and the Criminal Law, researcher and lecturer at the Faculty of Law at the Wolfgang-Goethe-Universität in Frankfurt (1978–1984, 1992–1993), the Faculty of Law and Economics at the Johannes-Gutenberg-Universität in Mainz (1984–1997). 1993 habilitation dissertation on the 'Market of Virtue'. Appointment to a full professorship (C4) for sociology at the Heinrich-Heine-Universität Düsseldorf in 1997. Main research areas: general sociological theory, rational choice theory, sociology of law, ethics and the social sciences. With Anton Leist he founded and still is editor of the journal Analyse und Kritik.
Heinrich-Heine-Universität, Sozialwissenschaftliches Institut, Lehrstuhl für Soziologie I, Germany

Breyer, Friedrich, Professor Dr. rer. pol., Dipl.-Volksw., study, doctorate and habilitation at the university of Heidelberg. 1986–92 professor at the Fern-Universität Hagen. Since 1992 professor of public economics at the Universität Konstanz; research professor at the Deutsche Institut für Wirtschaftsforschung, Berlin. Member of the Advisory Council of the German Ministry of Commerce. Research areas: health economics, social security.
Universität Konstanz, FB Wirtschaftswissenschaften, Konstanz, Germany

Fritze, Jürgen, Professor Dr. med., studied medicine at six German universities; 1975 final German exam and American (ECFMG) exam. 1978 Doctoral thesis on purification and characterization of brain dopamine receptors. 1979–1984 Specialization in Neurology and Psychiatry. 1985–1991 senior registrar at the Department of Psychiatry, University of Würzburg. Research on biological psychiatry. Since 1991 lecturer of psychiatry. 1991–1994 head of clinical research (phase I–IV) of Troponwerke (a Bayer subsidiary). 1994–1996 vice director of the Department of Psychiatry, University of Frankfurt. 1993–1999 Vice president of the German college of neuropsychopharmacology and pharmacopsychiatry (AGNP). Since 1997 Professor of Psychiatry. Since 1997 head of Medical Affairs of the German Association of Private Health Insurers. Editor of Psycho, member of the advisory board of various national and international journals. Main research: Psychopharmacology, molecular genetics, pharmacoeconomics, public health.
Verband der privaten Krankenversicherung, Köln, Germany

Hahn, Susanne, Dr. phil., studies of philosophy and history at the universities of Essen and Duisburg, 1992 Magister Artium at the University of Essen. 1998

Dr. phil. "Überlegungsgleichgewicht(e) – Prüfung einer Rechtfertigungsmetapher" [Reflective Equilibrium – Inquiry of a metaphor of justification], University of Essen. 1998–2000 collaborator of the project "Altersbezogene Rationierung von Gesundheitsleistungen im liberalen Rechtsstaat – Ethische, ökonomische und institutionelle Aspekte" [Age-based rationing in the liberal constitutional state – ethical, economical and institutional aspects] with H. Kliemt and F. Breyer, supported by the DFG. Since January 2001 scholarshipholder of a Lise-Meitner-Habilitationsstipendium. Main research areas: methodological approaches in practical and theoretical philosophy, rationing in medicine, constructivist philosophy (Nelson Goodman, Erlanger Schule), explication of rationality in game theory.
Gerhard-Mercator-Universität Duisburg, Fachbereich 1 – Philosophie, Germany

Hunter, David J., Professor of Health Policy and Management, studied political science at the University of Edinburgh, 1974 MA Hons (Soc. Sci.). Postgraduate studies at the University of Edinburgh. 1977 PhD. Professor of Health Policy and Management at the University of Durham (1999). Professor of Health Policy and Management, University of Leeds (1989–99). Director, Nuffield Institute for Health, University of Leeds (1989–97). Health policy analyst, King's Fund Institute, London (1987–89). Department of Community Medicine, University of Aberdeen (1982–1986). Health policy officer, Royal Institute of Public Administration, London (1980–82). Chair of the Health Development Group, University of Durham Business School (2001). Advisor to World Health Organisation (European Regional Office) on health sector reform (1989–). Member of the NHS Executive Northern and Yorkshire Regional Office's Modernisation Board (2000–) and its Task Board on Health Inequalities and Health Improvement (2001–). Chair of the Northern and Yorkshire Region's Public Health Observatory (2000–). Council member of the UK Public Health Association (2000–). Specialist advisor to the House of Commons Health Committee on its inquiry into the public health function (2000–2001). Member of the Health Development Agency's Policy Advisory Panel (2000–). Member of the NHS Managers' Group, AstraZeneca (1999–). Former Board Director and President of the European Health Management Association (1990– 1998). Former Non Executive Director, Leeds Health Authority (1990–1999). Main research areas: primary care, public health and health inequalities, managing clinical work, health care rationing.
University of Durham Business School, England

Imhoff, Michael, Dr. med., 1981–1987 study of human medicine at the universities of Bochum and Münster. 1988 dissertation at the Ruhr-University Bochum. 1991 Lederle Price for research on the application of time series analysis techniques to the monitoring of ICU patients. 1988–1994 resident at the Surgical Department, Community Hospital, Dortmund. 1994 board of surgery. Since 1994 senior surgeon and intensive care specialist, head of the surgical intensive care unit at Surgical Department, Community Hospital, Dortmund. 1996 board of surgical intensive care medicine. Since 1997 attending intensivist and head of the surgical intensive care unit, Community Hospital, Dortmund. Research in the fields of surgical intensive care medicine and computer applications in critical care. Collaborative Research Center with the Departments of Statistics and Informatics of the uni-

versity of Dortmund "Reduction of Complexity in multivariate Data Structures" (DFB Sonderforschungsbereich 475).
Städtische Kliniken Dortmund, Chirurgische Klinik, Dortmund, Germany

Kliemt, Hartmut, Professor Dr., degrees in management science and philosophy. After holding positions as research assistant in operations research, 1974–1976, and philosophy of law, 1976–1980, "Habilitation-Grant" and Habilitation at Frankfurt in 1983, afterwards temporary professorships in Munich and Frankfurt, full professor for practical philosophy at Duisburg since 1988. Adjunct research associate of The Center for Study of Public Choice in Fairfax, VA. Main interests are: applications of elementary game theory to basic problems of political theory, economic and ethical issues of health care, political philosophy in particular of the British Moralists.
Universität GH Duisburg, Fach Philosophie, Germany

Krämer, Walter, Professor Dr. rer. pol., studied Mathematics and Economics at the University of Mainz. Diploma in Mathematics 1976. PhD in Economics 1979. Lecturer at the University of Mannheim 1976–1980. Assistant Professor, University of Western Ontario (1980–1981), Vienna Institute for Advanced Studies (1982–1985), University of Hannover (1985–1988). Since 1988 Professor of Business and Economic Statistics, University of Dortmund. Since 1996 elected referee for statistics of the German Research Foundation (DFG). Research areas: health economics, capital markets, econometrics.
Universität Dortmund, Institut für Wirtschafts- und Sozialstatistik, Germany

Lübbe, Weyma, Professor Dr. phil. habil., studied philosphy, literature, sociology and economics at the universities of Zurich, Constance and Munich. 1984 M.A. in philosophy, 1989 Dr. phil., 1997 habilitation in philosophy. Research and teaching assistant in sociological and philosophical departments, 1988–1989 dissertation grant (Hanns Martin Schleyer Foundation), 1995–1996 habilitation grant (DFG – German Research Foundation), 1997–1998 fellow of the Institute for Advanced Studies (Berlin), 1998 Heisenberg grant (DFG), 1999 Rudolf Meimberg award (Academy for the Sciences and Literature, Mainz). Since 1999 full professor at the university of Leipzig. Main research areas: philosophy of law, applied ethics, history and epistemology of the social sciences.
Universität Leipzig, Philosophical Department, Germany

Raspe, Heiner, Professor, MD, PhD, Dr. med. et phil., works at the Medical University of Lübeck where he is Director of the Institute for Social Medicine. He is member of the Scientific Panel of the Council of Health Care Research for the Federal Ministry of Education, Science, Research and Technology. Since 1993 he has been vice president of the German Society for Social Medicine and Prevention. Member of the ethics commission of the State Board of Physicians and was a founding member of the Academy for Ethics in Medicine. His previous positions include Acting Director of the Department of Rheumatology at the Medical University, Hannover, elected member of the German Society for Rheumatology and resident expert in the fields of Medical Sociology and Social Medicine at the

Institute for Medical and Pharmaceutical Examination Questions. From 1990 to 1993, he was a speaker of the Commission Regional Rheumatological Care for the German Society of Rheumatology. Between 1991–1995, he was Chairman of the Standing Committee on Epidemiology at EULAR. Since 1997 speaker of the North German network of rehabilitation research, since 1998 speaker of the German network for Evidence-based Medicine. Main fields of work: Clinical, population-based and health care epidemiology, mainly of rheumatic diseases; rehabilitation research; evidence-based clinical Medicine and Health Care; Quality Management.
Institute for Social Medicine of the Medical University, Lübeck, Germany

Schöne-Seifert, Bettina, Dr. med. Dr. phil. habil., studied medicine at the universities of Freiburg, Göttingen, and Wien, Philosophy at the Georgetown University/Washington DC and again in Göttingen. 1982 doctoral thesis on the myelinization of rats with experimental phenylketonuria; 1984–1987 medical internship (Pediatric Hospital/Univerity of Göttingen); 1987 M.A. degree at Georgetown for philosophy/bioethics. Postdoctoral grant for medical ethics by the Stifterverband für die Deutsche Wissenschaft. 1990–1996 assistent professor for philosophy at the University of Göttingen. 1994–1995 fellow at the Center for Advanced Studies at Berlin. 1997–2000 scientist at the Center for Ethics/university of Zürich. 2000 Habilitation for philosophy at the university of Göttingen. Since 2001 visiting professor at the Center for Philosophy and Ethics of Science/university of Hannover. Member of the National Ethics Council. Main research interests: Medical ethics, applied ethics, ethical theory.
Zentrale Einrichtung für Wissenschaftstherorie und Wissenschaftsethik der Universität Hannover, Hannover, Germany

Schultheiss, Carlo, Dr. phil., M.A., studied philosophy, political science and German language and literature at the Universities of Freiburg and Konstanz. 1987 M.A. in philosophy and German language and literature (University of Konstanz). 1989 state exam in political science (University of Konstanz). 1990–1992 teacher training course. 1998 doctorate of social theory at the University of Leipzig (subject of the dissertation: methodological individualism/theory of rational choice). Since 1998 research assistant at the Faculty of Law, Economics and Politics of the University of Konstanz. Main research areas: social theory, biomedical ethics.
Universität Konstanz, Fachbereich Wirtschaftswissenschaften, Konstanz, Germany.

Szymkowiak, Christoph H., Dr. rer. nat., studied at Freie Universität Berlin. 1984 diploma, 1984–1987 doctorate at the Max-Planck Institut für molekulare Genetik. 1987–1990 researcher at UC Berkeley, Biochemistry Department, and at Stanford University, Department of Pathology. 1990–1995 researcher at Medizinische Universität zu Lübeck in the Department of Clinical Rheumatology. 1995–1998 Deutsches Zentrum für Luft- und Raumfahrt, working in a project management agency for government projects financed by the ministry of science and education and the ministry of health. 1998–2000 Verband der Angestellten Krankenkassen (VdAK),

currently employed by Techniker Krankenkassen (Substitute Sickness Fund), Department for Corporate Development.
Techniker Krankenkasse, Hamburg, Germany

Taupitz, Jochen, Prof. Dr., studied law in Göttingen and Freiburg. 1980 doctorate on problems of tort law. Senior research assistant at the University of Göttingen. 1988 post-doctoral thesis on "Professional Codes of Ethics". 1988 professor of law at the University of Göttingen. 1990 Chair of Civil Law, Civil Procedure Law, Private International Law and Comparative Law at the University of Mannheim. Further appointments to full professorships at the universities of Kiel (1993) and Bonn (1997). Publications on all fields mentioned and on medical law, public health law, credit card law and environmental law. Since 1996 part-time judge at the Higher Regional Court of Appeal (Oberlandesgericht) in Karlsruhe. Since 1998 Managing Director of the Institute for German, European and International Medical Law, Public Health Law and Bioethics of the Universities of Heidelberg and Mannheim. Since 2001 member of the National Ethics Advisory Board.
Universität Mannheim, Fakultät für Rechtswissenschaft, Lehrstuhl für Bürgerliches Recht, Zivilprozeßrecht, Internationales Privatrecht und Rechtsvergleichung.
Institut für Deutsches, Europäisches und Internationales Medizinrecht, Gesundheitsrecht und Bioethik der Universitäten Heidelberg und Mannheim; Lehrstuhl für Bürgerliches Recht, Zivilprozeßrecht, Internationales Privatrecht und Rechtsvergleichung, Germany

Thiele, Felix, M.D., M.Sc., has been Vice Director of the Europäische Akademie GmbH since 1999. He brings combined expertise in medicine and philosophy to this position. He studied medicine in Hamburg and Heidelberg and received an M.D. from the University of Heidelberg for an experimental work in the field of high blood pressure research. He furthermore received a Master of Science in Philosophy and History of Science from the London School of Economics. Before joining the academy he worked in the field of Science Management at the Max-Delbrueck-Center for Molecular Medicine Berlin Buch. At the academy he was manager of the project "Human Genetics. Ethical Problems and Societal Consequences" and is member of the study group "Practical Philosophy".
Europäische Akademie zur Erforschung von Folgen wissenschaftlich-technischer Entwicklungen Bad Neuenahr-Ahrweiler GmbH, Germany

Wambach, Achim, D.Phil., 1988–1991 studies of mathematics and physics at the university of Cologne, Germany. 1991–1994 D.Phil. in theoretical physics from Oxford University, UK. 1994–1995 Master of Science in Economics at the London School of Economics, UK, since then assistant professor at the university of Munich, Germany. 2000 habilitation for economics. Main research areas: Insurance economics, health economics, information economics, contract theory.
Department of Economics, University of Munich, Muenchen, Germany

Zweifel, Peter, Professor of Economics, 1969 diploma, 1974 doctoral degree from the University of Zurich. Honorary fellow at the University of Wisconsin in Madison. 1982 professorship ("An economic model of physician behavior"). Visiting professor to the University of the Armed Forces (Munich-Neubiberg), 1983 assistent professor at the university of Zurich, 1984 associate professor. Since 1990 full professor for economic theory and policy. Research interests in health economics, insurance economics, energy economics, and law and economics. Serves on the Swiss antitrust authority, the Competition Commission.

Socioeconomic Institute, University of Zurich, Switzerland

Contents

III Rationing, Ethics, and the Law

IV The Future of Rationing

Introduction

Friedrich Breyer, Hartmut Kliemt and Felix Thiele

"The Crisis of the Welfare State" has become a fashionable topic for research projects, academic conferences and political debates in recent decades. A quarter of a century after the emergence of the so-called "health-care cost explosion", there is a widespread belief that in the issue of health care financing the worst times are still ahead of us.

A recent estimate of the impact of demographic aging and technical progress in medicine on health care expenditures in Germany suggests that these two factors have the potential to raise the payroll tax necessary to finance sickness fund expenditures at the present conditions from 13.5 per cent today to over 23 per cent in 2040.[1]

Other branches of social insurance, in particular old-age pensions and long-term care will also become increasingly expensive as a result of population aging so that the total payroll tax burden, which is now at about 40 per cent in Germany (and which is held partly responsible for the high level of unemployment), might well reach 55 to 60 per cent if the present level of benefits is maintained. Nobody believes that it will be possible to place such an enormous burden on future working generations without risking their adverse reaction – be it through the political process or individually through a massive exit from official employment into the shadow economy or into countries with a less costly social safety net.

In line with the projections of future expenditure increases, the debate on how to contain this growth has intensified both in the political and the scientific arena. One of the main solutions proposed for averting the imminent health care crisis comes under the heading of "rationing" and thus – not surprisingly – the worldwide debate on whether and how to ration medical care has become very lively recently.

What is interesting, however, is that in the prevailing literature the concept of rationing itself has been far from unambiguous. In fact, several different notions of rationing are used, and this ambiguity has led to some misunderstandings.

There are essentially two kinds of ambiguities in the concept of rationing: The first ambiguity refers to the question whether rationing a good means *providing* the good to someone at less than its market price or *withholding* it from somebody. The second ambiguity refers to the question whether rationing is concerned with dividing a pie of given size (in which case rationing is primarily a matter of distributive justice) or with determining the size of the pie in a democratic society in a meaningful sense (in which case it has more to do with efficiency of allocation). In

---

[1] Cf. Breyer F and Ulrich V (2000), Gesundheitsausgaben, Alter und medizinischer Fortschritt: eine Regressionsanalyse. Jahrbücher für Nationalökonomie und Statistik 220, 1–17.

other words, is the need to ration a *consequence* of scarcity of health care resources or is rationing the act of allocating public resources to the health care sector and therefore the *cause* of the ensuing scarcity?

In the context of the crisis of the welfare state, it is the second meaning which is in our view increasingly important to address: what extent of medical services can society afford to provide within a collectively financed health system 30 years from now, and is it possible to solve the distributional problems involved in this decision along with the allocational ones as appropriately general "rule choices" from "behind the veil of ignorance", in other words: is it possible to avoid burdening physicians with answering the moral question "who shall live?" Whatever concept of rationing one favours, one should be aware of the fact that there are several concepts of rationing that should be kept apart carefully.

The present volume is the result of a conference devoted to the topic "Rationing in Medicine. Ethical, Legal and Practical Aspects", which was organized by the Europäische Akademie zur Erforschung von Folgen wissenschaftlich-technischer Entwicklungen and was held in Bad Neuenahr on March 23–25, 2000. It was one of the purposes of the organizers of the conference and the editors of this volume to contribute to a clarification of the concept of rationing and thereby help the participants in the debate to avoid further unnecessary confusion. Participants with a wide spectrum of knowledge, insight and experience were invited to contribute to the conference and the conference volume: academics from the disciplines of medicine, philosophy, economics and law as well as practitioners of health care itself and from the field of health-care financing.

The volume is organized in four sections. In Section I entitled *Rationing in international perspective*, the authors take stock in two ways: first, with respect to the concepts of rationing or, what is sometimes used synonymously, prioritising in health care, and secondly with respect to the practice of rationing in the country which figures prominently when practical examples of rationing are needed, the United Kingdom.

In Chapter 1, *Rationing: Distribution, Limitation, or Denial – Against Conceptual Confusion in the Debate about Health Care Systems*, Susanne Hahn points out several ambiguities of the concept of rationing as it is used in the debate – e.g., rationing as allocation and rationing as limitation. Hahn claims that the philosophical method of explication is the adequate method for pinning down the meaning of an already used term. After outlining the method of explication, she applies this method to the concept of rationing and concludes that not one single concept of rationing should be adopted, but more than one – relative to the aims (or interests of the speaker, as she calls it) pursued in using the concept of rationing.

Carlo Schultheiss in Chapter 2, *A Note on the Semantics of Rationing as Limitation*, also uses the method of explication for an investigation of concepts of rationing understood as limitation. He distinguishes three types of differences within the concept of rationing as limitation concerning, first, the standards relative to which health care is limited, second, concerning the normative presupposition invested in the term 'rationing', and thirdly, the levels of health care delivery on which limitation is effective. Finally Schultheiss points out several difficulties that these concepts are confronted with.

A clarification of the concept (or concepts) of rationing alone is not sufficient for actually implementing rationing in practice. Chapter 3 by Hans-Heiner Raspe on *Prioritizing and Rationing* discusses ways how to specify medically and morally acceptable criteria for rationing health services. Besides the conceptual difficulties in dealing with the concept of rationing, the actual practice of rationing is highly context-dependent, i.e. tied to the health care system in which rationing is practiced. This becomes clear in Chapter 4 by David Hunter on *The Practice of Rationing in Health Care in the United Kingdom*. Starting from an overview over the history of rationing in the British health care system, Hunter examines the question of whether – provided there is a scientifically sound method of adequate rationing – rationing can be implemented in a way leaving no problems unsolved or whether 'muddling through' is an essential feature of any feasible health care policy.

Interpreting Hunter as giving a pessimistic view on the chances of success of any rational (i.e., explicit, criteria driven) approach to rationing, Bettina Schöne-Seifert in Chapter 5, *Comment on David Hunter*, poses several questions that potentially weaken Hunter's claim for "elegantly muddling through": Would patients accept implicit rationing that is disguised as clinical judgement? Would the physician's self-understanding as the patient's advocate change? Would such a publicly financed health system resist the growing pressure for more individual choice? And finally, are philosophical concepts of justice in healthcare actually impracticable?

As we are convinced that rationing is practiced not only in the UK, but in a widespread manner, though often in concealed ways, Section II is devoted to the discussion of *Practices of Rationing in Germany*.

Against the background of growing health care expenditures the role of "high-tech" medicine has become of increasing interest. Though probably the single most resource consuming specialty in hospital care, there is according to Michael Imhoff a severe lack of work on the practices of rationing in intensive care. In Chapter 6, *Rationing in Intensive Care Medicine*, Imhoff aims at providing some empirically founded insights: A description of current practices of rationing is followed by some reflections on the role of the medical decision-making process in the context of rationing and a desired increase of cost-effectiveness.

Recently, global budgets have been advocated as adequate measures for controlling health care expenditure. Since the introduction of global budgets is controversially debated in Germany (and elsewhere), a panel discussion during the conference was devoted to the relation between global budgets and rationing. Chapter 7 reproduces the statements given by three of the participants – Walter Krämer, Peter Zweifel, Christof Szymkowiak – of this panel (Eckhard Nagel also participated in the discussion). A special focus lay on the moral relevance of whether statistical or individual lives are affected by rationing through budgeting procedures.

Section III – *Rationing, Ethics, and the Law* – discusses the present practice of rationing in the light of patient rights and of theories of distributive justice. In Chapter 8, Jochen Taupitz examines *The impact of the German Constitution on Rationing in Medicine*. The economic analysis of law, which gives financial effectiveness a great influence on the law-making process has been given increasing attention recently, so that the question arises to what extent the German constitution poses limits on rationing in medicine. Taupitz investigates whether the following rights can be derived from the German constitution: i) the right to specific health care services, ii) the right to non-discriminatory distribution of health services, and iii) the right to appropriate information of patients.

Presupposing that the health care system should be (at least partly) publicly organized and that medical resources are limited, Michael Baurmann deals in his contribution *Rationing Yes, Politics No. For a Right-based Approach in Rationing Medical Goods* (Chapter 9) with the role of the state in the pursuit of the ethical aims of health care provision. He differentiates and discusses two main focuses in allocating health care resources: *equality* (of access to health care) and *maximization* (of likely outcomes of health care). Viewing civil rights and rights to health care as parallel Baurmann supports the incorporation of rationing into the practice of health care since he believes that this is necessary to control the exercise of otherwise arbitrary power in the pursuit of the aim of maximizing the contribution of public health care to welfare.

The usage of different concepts of distributive justice as applied to the task of just allocation of health care resources is the topic of Weyma Lübbe's contribution (Chapter 10). Under the title *Rationing – Basic Philosophical Principles and the Practice* she investigates the ethical positions of utilitarianism, egalitarianism, and libertarianism; she examines the arguments in favour and against these concepts, their applicability to the practical problems of allocating scarce medical resources, and finally makes some remarks on the desirable as well as the likely future development of the rationing debate.

The final Section IV, *The Future of Rationing*, is concerned with a possible division of labor which might gain importance as soon as it is universally accepted that collectively financed health care systems can not provide all medically beneficial services at zero costs to every citizen: Is it possible that private insurance can provide financial access to additional services that are no longer covered by public financing schemes?

In Chapter 11, *Complementarity of Private and Public Insurance*, Jürgen Fritze provides some empirical data that may enlighten the debate on the question where and to what extent private insurance can substitute benefits that are up to now provided by the public insurance.

Likewise discussing the interplay of private and public insurance in Chapter 12, *Rationing of Health Care and the Complementarity of Private and Public Insurance*, Achim Wambach focuses on three interrelated questions. First, he examines why there should be public insurance at all. Second, he makes some remarks on what rules for rationing should be like from the perspective of economic theory. Finally, he turns to the question of how such a system of rationing might develop in practice.

The volume is concluded by Hartmut Kliemt's summary thoughts which he presented at the end of the conference. These originally spontaneous remarks were to a large extent provoked by the contributions and discussions at the conference and they are intended to provoke further thought.

I Rationing in international Perspective

Rationing: Distribution, Limitation, or Denial? – Against Conceptual Confusion in the Debate about Health Care Systems[1]

Susanne Hahn

1
'Rationing' – A Disturbing Concept

The term 'rationing' plays a central role within the political and scientific debates concerning the reform of health care systems. Sentences like "The demographical development accompanied by the progress in medicine makes rationing inevitable", "If we don't rationalize now we will have to ration in the near future", "A fixed budget of medical costs will result in rationing" are often heard in this political debate. The concept of rationing that is used in such statements clearly has negative connotations; the rationing of medical services is a threat.

The quarrel about the revision of health care systems as it is presented in the media is meanwhile accompanied by scientific reasoning. Economists, sociologists, philosophers, lawyers etc. investigate problems concerned with the rationing of health care services. In their investigations they use the term 'rationing' and related terms as 'is rationed' or 'someone rations' differently. The different usages – i.e. the different meanings – of the words are sometimes implicit, sometimes they are explicitly stated in definitions given.

The most widespread usage of the concept of rationing in the context of health care services is the use in a limiting sense: If someone rations health care services he limits these services. The kinds of limitation differ: some authors mean limitation below medical necessity, below a level of medical benefit or limitation compared with the hitherto provided services in the health care insurance. Authors who strongly oppose the limitation of publicly funded health care services often stress the aspect of limitation by defining rationing as the denial of services or goods. Especially in response to this interpretation some authors point out that the term 'rationing' is not a new term which is only used in the debate about health care reform. On the contrary it is a notion with a well defined meaning in the politics of economics. This usage of rationing means the distribution or allocation of goods or services and not their denial. If someone, or better, if the state rations goods, it distributes these goods.

[1]   The paper is part of a research project supported by the DFG (KL-480/5-1).

Summing up one can distinguish two sorts of usages of the expression 'rationing': While usages of the first sort stress the aspect of limitation as being essential for rationing, usages of the second sort stress the public allocation of goods. Therefore one has to state the ambiguity of the term.

Why is it so important to avoid ambiguities? Consider the phrase: "The rationing of health care services is justified". In the allocating sense it would mean: "The administrative allocation of health care services is justified". In the limitating sense it would mean: "The limitation of health care services is justified" or stronger: "The denial of health care services is justified". Thus the phrase "The rationing of health care services is justified" can express completely incongruent positions. At first glance different people who utter the same phrase seem to be in perfect harmony but on the second glance they completely disagree. The misunderstandings cannot be broached by refering to the context because the context remains the same: the debate about health care reform. So it is not a trivial ambiguity as in the examples "poach" and "ounce": If someone utters "I will poach an egg" it is clear that he will not go illegally into the forest to shoot an egg, but will simmer it in water. It will also cause no confusion if someone describes a person with the phrase: "He has eyes like an ounce". The context makes sure that he does not mean the measurement but the animal.

The risks involved in ambiguity and the importance of a definite meaning for the treatment of a problem, make it necessary to care for the concise usage: The adequate method to fix the meaning of an already used term is the method of explication as it was developed by Carnap and Quine.

2
Some Remarks on Explication

By means of explication the meaning of an already used expression is fixed. Candidates for an explication are on the one hand ambiguous terms, whose ambiguity cannot be solved refering to the context and on the other side vague expressions. Examples for the ›trivial‹ ambiguities are the mentioned verb 'poach' and the noun 'ounce'. In these cases the reference to a context solves the ambiguity so that there is no need for an explication.

But there are also ›risky‹ ambiguous uses of expressions that cannot be made definite by referring to the context. An example for this kind is the term 'conclusion': Using this noun an author can mean a conclusion scheme, a particular inference out of certain premises or the derived proposition. The context is always the same: a scenario of logical deduction. The use of 'conclusion' does not become clear cut in this context. To obtain unequivocal usage one has to give an explication.

Another reason for giving an explication are vague concepts. Similar to the ambiguous expressions one has to distinguish harmless and risky cases. Harmless are those cases in which there is no or no high liability in connection with the usage of a vague expression. For example if someone describes a person to be met at the station as tall, blond etc. In most cases it will not be necessary to give a definition of 'tall' in centimeters. On the other hand if such a measure gets binding as for example in laws one has to make sure a definite use. The obligation to chain up tall dogs is vague insofar there are dogs of middle measure so that it is not clear if they are already tall or still small. In these obligatory matters there is need for explication, in this case fulfilled by giving a precise measure for the tallness of dogs.

The method of explication covers a descriptive and a normative part.[2] Descriptively the different usages of an expression are found out and listed. In the mentioned example one would have to list the various meanings of 'conclusion'. To fulfill the descriptive part one also has to state the synonyms if there are any.

On the basis of this description of usage the normative part is carried out. Firstly the *explicandum* has to be determined. Thereby *one* desirable usage of the term is pointed out. For example one could point out as the explicandum of 'conclusion' the usage as the derived proposition. The purpose of an explication is to regulate the term so that its meaning is fixed by a definition or another mode of determining usage.

Aiming at being able to decide if an explication is adequate one has to establish a *measure of explication* in advance. It consists of propositions which have to be decidable – among others – by the explicat given. In the example it could contain the proposition 'If A is the conclusion of a deduction there is a class of premises P and a set of rules R so that A is derived out of P applicating some r out of R'. – An explication is adequate if the statements of the measure of explication are decidable. Otherwise, the explication is inadequate. In that case the measure of explication has to be changed or the explication itself, i.e. the fixing of the desired usage.

Explications are characterized by regulating the future usage of terms already used. Such regulations are not limited to scientific languages. Rather they are found in all those areas in which there are strong interests to distinguish. Various legal norms represent examples: 'Murder', 'employee', 'contributable' are terms whose usage is determined by respective rules or other procedures with equivalent perfomance.

3
Different Meanings of 'Rationing'

In the introduction the term 'rationing' was characterized as ambiguous and therefore in need of explication. Applicating the method of explication one has to ask: Which usages have to be distinguished?

3.1
The Usage in the Tradition of Economic Policy

Participants in the debate on health care reform rejecting the interpretation of rationing as a denial, point out that traditionally and with respect to other sorts of goods rationing means something different.

---

[2] The presented account of the method of explication stands in the tradition of Carnap and Quine. Their approach is elaborated e.g. in Siegwart, Explikation. Further literature is also given there.

The notion of rationing is not a new one, but stems from times of scarcity, e.g. times of war and post-war. The rationing of food or energy are typical examples for rationed goods in these periods of need. In these contexts the speech of rationing is mostly done by the use of the predicate 'is rationed': "Bread and butter are rationed".

"Vahlens Großes Wirtschaftslexikon" (an economic lexicon) characterizes rationing as:

> behördliche Zuteilung von Gütern (Bewirtschaftung); wird vor allem in Krisensituationen (Krieg etc.) eingeführt und ersetzt den Markt als Zuteilungsmechanismus durch administrative Anordnung.[3]
> (the official distribution of goods which is carried out especially in times of crises and which replaces the market as the distributing mechanism by implementing administrative allocation.)

The essential characteristics for rationing are *the annulment of the market for goods and its replacement by an official allocation*. The institution that annuls the market and takes over the distribution of goods is in most cases the state. The reason for taking this step is the scarcity of a sort of goods and the scenario that is caused thereby: The supply, being too small in relation to demand, causes rising prices. The high prices make it impossible for some or most potential consumers to buy these goods.[4] However, there would still be enough buyers of the goods at high prices who would clear the market. Therefore the – hypothetical – prices can be characterized as clearing the market.

Hence rationed goods are offered below market clearing prices. Summed up in a definition by Kliemt:

> Rationierung ist ein Vorgang, in dem bestimmte Dienstleistungen oder Güter bestimmten Personen in festen Quantitäten unterhalb markträumender Preise zugänglich gemacht werden.[5]
> (Rationing is a process that makes certain services or goods accessible to certain persons in fixed quantities below market clearing prices.)

The described situation of scarcity accompanied by rising prices does not automatically cause a regulated allocation. Small harvests in Bordelais entailing a rise of prices of 50 per cent per bottle does not motivate any state to assure every citizen the supply with *cru*-wines.

Another condition has to be fulfilled for the rationing of goods: The supply with these goods must be judged as a public interest. This does not apply with Bordeaux-wines. At least up to now they are not judged as elementary. On the other hand food products as for example bread, water and rice are seen as goods being absolutely necessary for human nutrition so that one has to assure the supply with these.

In sum the depicted usage of 'is rationed' stresses the aspect of allocation: There is an *allocating* institution, an *allocated* good and someone who *receives* a good. The mentioning of a process and the reference to market clearing prices refer to a

---

[3]   Vahlens Großes Wirtschaftslexikon, p 1776.
[4]   Vahlens Großes Wirtschaftslexikon mentions social deliberations as main reason for the rationing of elementary goods; cf. Vahlens Großes Wirtschaftslexikon, p 1776.
[5]   Kliemt, Gesundheitsversorgung bei Ressourcenknappheit – Ethische Aspekte, p 110.

parameter of time with respect to a sequence of states. Characterizing a situation as a situation of rationing means to refer to a different state before. More precisely: One compares a situation in which the goods of a certain sort are allocated by the market with a situation in which these goods are allocated by a public institution.

An informal reconstruction of this traditional usage of the concept of rationing taking into account the time parameter and the aspect of market clearing prices runs as follows:

R1 x rations y towards z at t
iff
x is a sovereign body and y is an elementary good for z and t is some point in time and the distribution of y before t is performed by market procedures and from t on it holds: there is a finite quantity n and the selling price of y after t is less than the market price of y before t and x allocates y to z in the quantity n.

The definition contains the four aspects that are essential for this usage of the term 'rationing': the allocating sovereign, the receiving counterpart, the elementary allocated good and the change of the situation of consumption from a certain point in time.

Parties in the debate about health care reform who point out this traditional use of rationing want to make clear that in the first place health services are allocated and not withheld as the opponents to limited health care suppose. Their suggestion could be seen as the attempt to free the notion of rationing from its completely negative connotations. For the same reason some of the American authors prefer to use the term allocation instead of rationing.

3.2
Rationing in the Debate about Health Care Reform

The usage of the concept of rationing in the debates about health care reform *differs* in most cases *essentially*. To ration health care services simply means to limit them. Many opponents of rationing understand the rationing of health care services even more rigorously as a denial: "Gesundheitsleistungen rationieren bedeutet, Patienten eine wirksame Behandlung vorzuenthalten."[6] (To ration health care services means to deny the patients an effective treatment.) Statements that interpret rationing as a supply below the medically necessary seem to point into a similar direction: "Rationierung bedeutet, daß bestimmte medizinisch sinnvolle und verfügbare Versorgungsangebote aus dem Leistungskatalog der GKV gestrichen werden."[7] (Rationing means to remove certain beneficial and disposable offers of supply from the catalogue of services provided by the public health care insurance.)

The widespread indignation that accompanies every statement, stressing the need of the rationing of health care services, suggests that the following connection

---

[6] Smith, Plädoyer für eine offene Rationierungsdebatte, p 2453; see also Kühn who suspects capitalistic ideology and socially selective systems with all kind of denial of health care services: Kühn, Rationierende Medizin: Praxis und Ideologie der "Rationierung" in den USA und Großbritannien, pp 65–67.

[7] Mielck/John, Kostendämpfung im Gesundheitswesen durch Rationierung – Was spricht dafür und was dagegen?, p 2.

is subsumed: The ›good‹ health is of such an enormous importance that all measures serving the maintenance of health or its recovery have to be delivered or funded publicly.

Similar to the usage in the economic sense it is obvious that the usage of 'rationing' in the above mentioned sense also relates two different states: The state in which health care services are rationed, i.e. limited, is distinguished from a state in which these services are distributed in accordance with the need of those who get them.

The widespread usage of 'rationing' in the limiting sense conceals this comparative respect. Nevertheless, it is just its revelation that makes it possible to explain why the rationing of services is meant to be a limitation and therefore to explain the indignation in view of this state of affair.

The delineated usage in its limiting or withholding interpretation is also to reconstruct. The reconstruction refers to the most severe formulation of the limiting sense, the denial of medical services.

R2 x rations y towards z at t
      iff
      x is a medical sovereign body and y is an elementary medical good for z and x allocates y to z before t and from t onward x withholds y from z

The characterization of the limiting interpretation contains four aspects: the allocated or withheld good, the authority which allocates or withholds, the (non-)receiving counter-part, and the instance at which the situation of distribution changes. The medical sovereign stands vicariously for those allocating institutions that can also cooperate: state, insurance or physician.

3.3
'Rationing' – Further Usages

The inquiry of the usages of 'rationing' and related expressions has revealed an ambiguity in at least two respects. Besides these usages one can distinguish – at least – two further usages: The first one is a transfer of the distributing interpretation to the private domain. An example: One can speak of the rationing of a special wine if the wine-cellar sells each client only a limited number of the bottles in great demand, assuring that other clients will also get something. This usage of the concept of rationing differs in several respects from the distributing interpretation: It is doubtful that the good is elementary for a widespread range of receivers. In this case only clients are to be served, the cellar is rather a selling than an allocating institution and does not distribute a good in a certain number but fixes a maximum a client can buy. In sum, the concept of rationing is used just – rather unspecifically – in the sense of limited sale.

R3 x rations y towards z
      iff
      x is seller and z is buyer and there is a finite number n and x sells y to z in the maximum number n

To speak of the rationing of sweets or allowed times of television in family affairs represents further examples of this unspecific usage. In the definition above one has to substitute 'x is seller' by 'x is in possession of y and x has the power to decide regarding y' and 'z is buyer' by 'z is interested in y', 'x sells y to z' by 'x gives y to z'. The result of this substitution is: 'x rations y towards z iff x is in possession of y and x has the power to decide regarding y and z is interested in y and there is a finite number n and x gives y to z at the maximum number n.'

Another usage of 'rationing' proposes to regard goods even then as rationed – in a wider sense – if they have a price.[8] Following this interpretation nearly all goods were rationed. Exceptions could be freely accessible ›natural resources‹ as for example mushrooms, woodstrawberries and so on. Presupposing this usage one can only distinguish goods that have a price from those which have not. Further interests of distinguishing, being the reason for conceptual construction, cannot be pursued by a concept with such a high degree of generality. The distributing sense of rationing describes the circumstance that goods are allocated by a distributing institution in a finite number at fixed prices. For this state of affairs different expressions are needed and must be distinguished from a conception of rationing with this wide range of application.

3.4
Desired Usage – Determination of the Explicandum

The two last mentioned meanings are not relevant for the purpose at issue, i.e. the standardization of the rationing concept in the context of health care. Therefore they are no explicanda. The first usage is too unspecific as it pays neither attention to the aspect of distribution or limitation. The second usage does not promote the pursued object: Without further determinations it is not possible to distinguish between a state in which a sort of goods is freely purchasable and a state later on in which these goods are allocated below the market price; the goods are rationed in both cases.

With respect to the debate about health care reform the other two meanings of rationing that have been reconstructed by (quasi-)definitions are relevant: rationing in the distributing and in the limiting sense. They are candidates for the explicandum. But the potential explicanda differ considerably. The problem which meaning is intended is not solvable by reference to the context as it is possible with the examples 'poach' and 'ounce'. In the case at hand the context remains the same, the debate about health care reform. Moreover, the interpretations are not mutually substitutable.

The non-replaceability of the usages is shown in three steps: Firstly the limitating interpretation, being widespread in the health care system is generalized (i); secondly the distributing economic unterstanding is specialized with regard to the health care system (ii). Finally it is shown that the limiting reading cannot be integrated into the distributing interpretation (iii).

(i)   The distributing interpretation of rationing is not substitutable by the limiting interpretation

---

8   Cf. Breyer/Kliemt, Lebensverlängernde medizinische Leistungen als Clubgüter?, pp 132f.

Substituting the medical sovereign by the allocating sovereign and the elementary medical good by elementary goods of all sorts one gets:

R4 x rations y towards z at t
        iff
        x is an allocating sovereign body and y is an elementary good for z and x allocates y to z before t and from t onward x withholds y from z

The transfer of the limitating sense of rationing in the health care system to general affairs of rationing fails to meet the intuition of the distributing sense of rationing in several respects: *Firstly* – and most importantly – the idea of assuring the supply with goods judged sufficiently essential is obstructed: From an instant onward the goods are no longer distributed but simply withheld. One may raise an argument against, pointing to the fact that in circumstances of emergency goods that have been provided before are no longer supplied or are provided in smaller amounts. But one has to object that in those circumstances this *change* is not described as rationing but as a suspension of supply or a switch to smaller amounts of provision. *Secondly* the respect which is most essential for the distributing economic sense of rationing is dismissed: the substitution of market mechanisms by other procedures of distribution.

(ii)   The limitating interpretation of rationing is not substitutable by the distributing interpretation

Specializing the definition of the distributing interpretation to the domain of health care systems one gets:

R5 x rations y towards z at t in the health care system
        iff
        x is a medical sovereign body and y is an elementary medical good for z and t is some point in time and the distribution of y before t is performed by market procedures and from t on it holds: there is a finite quantity n and the selling price of y after t is less than the market price of y before t and x allocates y to z in the quantity n.

Firstly, this usage of the expression '..rations..towards..at..' stressing the allocating aspect cannot make plausible the highly negative connotations associated with the concept of rationing in health care. The threat of the utterance "If we get a global budget for the expenditures in the health care system then we have to ration the medicaments and the medical treatment" is only explainable presupposing a limitating interpretation of rationing. *Secondly*, the essential aspect of the distributing rationing, i.e. the substitution of the market by regulated allocation does not apply to the health care system. The debate about health care reform is just held in those states which already provide medical services publicly and not completely by market procedures.

(iii)   The limitating interpretation of rationing cannot be integrated into the distributing interpretation

The situation in which goods are rationed is partly associated with queuing and rations being always too small. Therefore one could propose to see limitation and distribution as reverse sides of the medal. Rationed goods are distributed, but not in the necessary measure; the distributed ration is seen as limited. A reconstruction of this approach could read as follows:

R6 x rations y towards z at t in the health care system
iff
x is a medical sovereign body and y is an elementary medical good for z and t is some point in time and the distribution of y before t is performed by market procedures and from t on it holds: there is a finite quantity n_1 and there is a finite quantity n_2 and n_1 is smaller than n_2 and the selling price of y after t is less than the market price of y before t and x allocates y to z in the quantity n_1.

Four arguments hold against this proposal:

Firstly: The definition catches the limitational character of the distribution, but not the aspect of withholding. Speaking of the denial of goods on the other hand presupposes a claim to the respective good: If someone withholds something to someone, then the latter has a claim to the withheld matter. The last definition includes the withholding effect only if one supposes that everyone has a claim to the amount of those goods he needs. Generally, only few goods are deemed to be so important that a claim of supply with this good is conceded to every individual or every citizen. As a rule, claims of this sort are not explicitly regulated but are the result of implicit societal processes. Summing up one has to state that the definition R6 does not regard or cannot regard the aspect of withholding being of great importance in the debate about health care systems.

Secondly: If one integrates the aspect of the denial of goods into the definition of rationing in the distributing sense, then the intention to assure the supply with a good by the method of rationing is obstructed: Those who annul the market to make sure that all potential consignees will be supplied do not withhold the respective goods.

Thirdly: The circumstance that market procedures are replaced does not apply to the health care system. Medical services are publicly funded and allocated in those health care systems being the object of reform.

Fourthly: In spite of including the aspect of allocation the definition does not comprehend the comparison between two situations of allocation: one in which the whole demand is supplied by allocation and one in which only a part of the demand is satisfied.

As an interim result it has to be recorded: In dealing with medical goods and services two aspects are virulent: On the one hand the public supply of goods and on the other hand their limitation, regarded as denial. – Presenting this result the inquiry of the ambiguity of the term 'rationing' is finished. The somewhat surprising result of this investigation does not consist in one explicandum, but in two.

3.5
Interests of Speech – Establishing a Measure of Explication

The essentially different usages pose a problem: Which meaning of the expression is to be fixed as the standard meaning by an explication? This question can only be answered referring to the interests of speech associated with the expression. Within the procedure of explication these interests are considered by establishing a measure of explication. A measure consists of those propositions that should be provable or refutable after having explicated the respective term. Therefore, the next step is to determine such propositions.

Taking into account the contributions to the debate about health care reform one ascertains three aspects in dealing with medical services that should become an issue of scientifical, philosophical and societal judgement: First, one can ask if the public allocation of medical services is desirable or justifiable. Furthermore, the most often posed question in the actual debate aims at the problem if the limitation of publicly funded medical services is justifiable. Finally one has to mention the problem of withholding medical services. – So, the following propositions should be decidable, i.e. provable or refutable, in a system reconstructed respectively:

(1) It is justified to allocate medical services publicly.
(2) It is justified to allocate medical services below a standard of medical necessity.
(3) It is justified to withhold medical services.

Thus far all of the three interests of speech are served by the concept of rationing. This circumstance is responsible – at least partly – for misinterpretations and pseudo-controversies: An affirmative answer to the question, if one is allowed to ration medical services has different meanings depending on the meaning of rationing. In the limitational sense of rationing it means that the rations of medical services may be smaller than the amount that are needed or – more rigorous – may be below the amount to which a claim exists. In the distributing sense of rationing an affirmative answer to the question means that medical services are judged to be so essential that they should be provided publicly, i.e. by measures of redistribution. For illustration:

It is justified: x rations y towards z at t
distributing sense

It is justified:
x is a medical sovereign body and
y is an elementary good for z and
t is some point in time and the
distribution of y before t is performed
by market procedures and from t on it
holds: there is a finite quantity n and
the selling price of y after t is less
than the market price of y before t and
x allocates y to z in the quantity n.

limitational sense

x is a medical sovereign body and
y is an elementary medical good for z
and x allocates y to z before t and from
t onward x withholds y from z.

Obviously, the different interests of speech *cannot* be satisfied employing *one* expression. As all three mentioned aspects with regard to the dealing with medical services should be attended to, one has to provide an unambigous description for the three circumstances. First, it is proposed to select the terms 'limitation' and 'denial' instead of a limitating and withholding interpretation of rationing. Further, one has to investigate in how far the distributing interpretation which is used in many contexts is transferable to the system of health care in the sense of proposition (1).

Two aspects of the distributing interpretation of rationing speak against the transfer to the (German) health care system: (i) the speech of fixed amounts of the allocated goods and (ii) the temporally and quantitatively comparing speech of states.

(i) The goods allocated in a health care system are more or less medical services. These are not distributed to every insured person or every citizen, but only to specific persons, i.e. to those that have been diagnosed by legitimated professionals to have a need of such goods. Therefore, it does not hold that every person gets a fixed amount of a good.

Approximating the interpretation of rationing in health care one could speak of the fixed amount of a claim, instead of the fixed amount of a good. The receiver would get an insurance of a certain size to a price below the market price. But the latter condition does not apply to all cases in a compulsory health care system:

The market prices of insurances are fixed with respect to the insured risk. Within a free insurance market persons with a low risk of getting ill have to pay less than risky persons. In publicly funded health care systems, intending to assure the supply with medical services for all, the prices for insurances are not set with regard to the risk of getting ill but for example with regard to incomes. In a compulsory health insurance system persons with high income and low risk of getting ill therefore pay prices beyond the market price and not below the market price.

(ii) The traditional characterization of rationed goods presupposes that there is a state before an instant in time t, in which goods of a certain sort are sold and bought on a free market and a state later on in which these goods are allocated by a public authority. This definition cannot be transferred to the present health care system. As medical services are allocated by a public health care system one cannot distinguish a state with a free market and a state with authoritative allocation.

In sum, one has to state the following result, which is quite astonishing regarding the initial aim of explication: If one wants to pose the question if medical services are goods of such an essential category that the supply with it is assured by public authorities one should – for the sake of unambiguity – not use the concept of rationing. On the contrary one has to assign other, not misleading terms for this purpose. Apart from assuring unambiguity this procedure has another advantage: It avoids the emotive meaning or "Sinnfärbung" (using a term of Gottlob Frege) of the concept of rationing. This emotive meaning is an obstacle in leading a matter-of-fact debate. By replacing the expression 'rationing' with words that elucidate the interests of speech unmistakably and without wide ranging connotations promotes the rational settling of the controversy.[9]

At this point, one may raise the objection that this strategy aims at a reform of language which will ultimately be impossible. The following remarks are in place: *For the present* this estimation applies insofar as scientific analysis cannot really change the usage of expressions in daily politics. Those taking part in the debate will presumably continue to speak of rationed medical services. Nevertheless, it will be necessary to distinguish at least the above mentioned matters discussing and deciding concrete fundamental health care reforms. If the parties taking part in the debate bring forward their concerns using the ambiguous concept of rationing, the different interests will make it indispensible to render the supposed meaning precise.

---

[9]　It is remarkable that this strategy encounters more refusal than sympathy. It seems as if all parties are interested in using the concept of rationing for specific interests – whatever they are.

In addition, a *scientific* discussion has of course to fulfill the following claims: It has to avoid obvious conceptual confusions or those having been made obvious that cause the confusions of the matters themself. Besides it has to eliminate those confusions that have occured already. Explications exactly fulfill this purpose; therefore it is not astonishing if they end with normative determinations. On the contrary, they are the aimed at and expectable results of explicational effort.

4
Subsequent Problems: Public Distribution and Denial of Medical Services

Which is the next step to be taken in order to provide a conceptual basis for dealing with problems of public health care systems? First of all those expressions have to be determined that should be introduced into a language used to treat respective questions. If these expressions are already used, one has to give an explicative introduction. If they are new, the introduction is "novative", i.e. it is not orientated along existing usages. – For the distributing interpretation of rationing the introduction of the 3-place predicate '..distributes..publicly to..' may be suitable.

How can the aspect of limitation be specified further? Without adding a specification, the limitation of the public allocation of medical services could mean the limitation to those measures which are medically necessary. It can as well mean the limitation to a level below medical necessity; an example could be the limitation of medical services with respect to the age of the patients. – Therefore, in order to decide the justifiability of limitating medical services it is not sufficient to speak generally of limitation. On the contrary, one first has to specify the catalogue of publicly funded or provided measures in question or one has to give a standard of limitation.

In addition, it is remarkable that the question of limitation arises only after having responded affirmatively to the first mentioned question: Those who reject the public allocation of medical services need not explain the position regarding the extent of services. On the contrary, those who affirm a public health care system are confronted with the question of its extend.

Regarding the denial of goods medical services do not differ from other services. The explicating part of the explicandum '..withholds..from..' contains as a constitutive part the claim to a service towards an institution. An explicative definition could run as follows: x withholds y to z iff x disposes of y and z has a claim to y towards x and x does not give y to z. – Definitions are correct if all expressions of the *definiens* are expressions already introduced. So, for the correctness of the mentioned definition it is essential that for example the usage of the expression '..has a claim to..towards..' is already ruled.

Apart from this task one can fix the following correlation: If one supposes a usage of denied goods as sketched above, and additionally supposes an obvious usage of 'is justified' and 'is unjustified', then one has to conclude that a denial of goods is by no means justified. Transferred to the debate about health care systems: Those who say that to ration medical services means to deny them need not raise the question of justifiability; they have already answered it. Using the vocabulary of denial is equivalent to presuppose a claim to medical services. Not to satisfy these claims means to act in an unjustified way. Proponents of this position do not take part in the discussion concerning the question "Are medical services or goods so essential and elementary that they should be provided by the public? And if this is so, to what extent should they be provided?". On the contrary, they presuppose a respective claim without further investigation.

To decide if an institution or a person withholds something to someone the specification of the claim is absolutely necessary. To assign the predicate '..with-holds..to..' to a state of affair is only possible after having specified the pertinent rights further. An affirmative answer to the question of publicly provided health care services is presupposed.

The disclosed correlation between denial and claim enables a judgement concerning the question of budgets in health care systems: If the health care system constitutes a claim to medical goods and services it is most unlikely that the ful-fillment of these claims is compatible with a practice of budgeting. Budgets make it necessary to save services. Therefore there will be patients who have a claim to certain services but do not get them, the services are withheld to them.

5
Conclusion: Well Constructed Conceptions for Methodological Problem Solving

The reconstruction of the speech of rationing in the debate on health care services disclosed risky ambiguities. Besides, it was found out that three of the ascertained usages touch essential concerns of allocating health care services publicly. Finally special features of the (public) health care system in Germany tell against an adoption of the meaning of rationing in a distributing sense as it is used in many domains. Therefore, in sum it is indicated to refrain from fixing one usage as an explicandum, determining its meaning by an explication. Rather the different interests of speech have to be recognized by – novative or explicative – intro-duction of respective different expressions. Regarding the context of health care some relations between public allocation, limitation and denial have been exposed.

Against those who assign the predicate of superfluousness to the whole project of explicating and constructing an unambiguous language as a basis of a rational debate – e. g. by pointing out that everyone knows what is meant if someone utters that the Big Macs have to be rationed in the future – one should object: These domains of acting and speaking, proceeding well without disturbances, are not the object of normative regulation. In these cases a reform of the use of language would actually be superfluous. But measures are not superfluous pure and simple, but superfluous in relation to pursued objects. If justifications or arguments must be put forward, as it is the case in the supposed context, the unambiguity of speech is not only not superfluous but a necessary prerequisite for a success of the respective issue of justification.

In all contexts dealing with terminological determinations and in all cases which are characterized by controversies, pseudo-dissents and pseudo-consents caused by differently used words, methodological efforts to assure the unambiguous use of the pertinent expressions are unavoidable. (At least) This is the contribution of philosophy to moral controversies. The slogan "Back to the relevant matters" often is issued when one has been caught in confusions lying far away from the ›relevant matters‹.

6
References

Breyer F, Kliemt H, Lebensverlängernde medizinische Leistungen als Clubgüter? In: Homann K (Hrsg.): Wirtschaftsethische Perspektiven I. Theorie, Ordnungsfragen, Internationale Institutionen, pp 131–158

Kliemt H (1997) Optimal Rationing – The Price of Value in Health Care. In: Dohrmann P, Henne-Bruns D, Kremer B: Surgical Efficiency and Economy, Proceedings of the 3rd World-Conference, Stuttgart-New York, pp 26–30

Kliemt H (1998) Gesundheitsversorgung bei Ressourcenknappheit – Ethische Aspekte. In: Nagel E, Fuchs Chr (Hrsg.) Rationalisierung und Rationierung im deutschen Gesundheitswesen, Stuttgart-New York, pp 109–114

Kühn H (1998) Rationierende Medizin: Praxis und Ideologie der "Rationierung" in den USA und Großbritannien. In: Kaupen-Haas H, Rothmaler Chr (Hrsg.) Strategien der Gesundheitsökonomie, Sozialhygiene und Public Health, Bd. 4, Frankfurt a.M., pp 65–86

Mielck A, John J (1996) Kostendämpfung im Gesundheitswesen durch Rationierung – Was spricht dafür und was dagegen? In: Gesundheitswesen 58, pp 1–9

Nagel E, Fuchs Chr (Hrsg.) (1998) Rationalisierung und Rationierung im deutschen Gesundheitswesen, Stuttgart-New York

Rebscher H (1998) Rationalisierung und Rationierung aus Sicht der Krankenversicherung. In: Nagel E, Fuchs Chr (Hrsg.) Rationalisierung und Rationierung im deutschen Gesundheitswesen, Stuttgart-New York, pp 27–41

Siegwart G (1997) Explikation. Ein methodologischer Versuch. In: Löffler W, Runggaldier E (Hrsg.) Dialog und System. Otto Muck zum 65. Geburtstag, Sankt Augustin, pp 15–45

Smith R, Plädoyer für eine offene Rationierungsdebatte. In: Deutsches Ärzteblatt 95 (1998), A-24534-2458 [Heft 40]

Vahlens Grosses Wirtschaftlexikon, hg. v. Dichtl E, Issing O, München 1993

A Note on the Semantics of Rationing as Limitation[1]

Carlo Schultheiss

1
Introduction

A wider public debate on the "rationing" of health care is called for repeatedly.[2] Such a debate is hindered by disagreement on the adequate use of the term "rationing". We can hardly hope for a fruitful wide debate as long as many participants use it in substantially different ways and as long as the disagreement on the adequate use of that term leads to contradictory answers to the question as to whether rationing really occurs in the health care systems in question.

To begin with, the current debates suffer from the fact that there is an *allocational* and a *limitational* concept of rationing.[3] According to the former concept, "rationing" simply means a process by which goods or services are made accessible in fixed quantities at prices below their market clearing prices (Kliemt 1998). Apparently, this definition serves to eliminate the negative connotations that are notoriously attached to that term. On the other hand most participants seem to prefer the limitational concept of rationing – that is a concept according to which rationing (by definition) limits the access to certain medical goods or services. Looked at more closely, this concept itself covers different meanings of what is called "rationing of health care".

The following remarks concentrate on the limitational concept and are guided by the philosophical method of explication. The first step of the procedure called "explication" consists (1) in listing different usages of the term that is to be explicated (and eventually in listing synonyms) and (2) in a specification of that meaning that is relevant for explication.[4] My examination belongs to this step of explication. Its first part offers a systematization of the alternative uses within the limitational concept. The second part points to some problems of definitions which can be regarded as examples of this concept and could in this way help to find the relevant explicandum.

---

[1] The article has been written for the project "Age-based rationing of health care in the liberal constitutional state – ethical, economic and institutional aspects" supported by the Deutsche Forschungsgemeinschaft (BR 740/13-1).
[2] See for example Smith (1998).
[3] See Hahn's contribution to this volume.
[4] See Siegwart (1997) and Hahn's comments on explication in the present volume.

2
Differences within the Limitational Concept of Rationing

According to the proposed systematization, there are at least three types of differences within the limitational concept. First, there are differences concerning the standard of limitation, second, there are differences concerning the evaluation of the policy termed "rationing". Third, we find differences with respect to the levels upon which decisions concerning the limitation of health care can be made.

2.1
Differences Concerning the Standard of Limitation

Some proponents of the limitational concept of rationing – for whatever reasons – do not specify the standard of limitation. Rebscher (1998) for example characterizes rationing as a "quantitative limitation of health care services". This means that in the case of rationing, patients receive less than a certain amount N, but among those who define the phrase in a more precise manner there is no consensus on the measures for the determination of N.

One point of view maintains that the "medically necessary goods or services" should be regarded as the reference point of limitation. Thus, Hadorn and Brook (1991) suppose that "care duly deemed necessary" – as opposed to merely effective, appropriate, or beneficial services – is the most adequate standard of limitation. Moreover, they believe that panels of experts should determine which services have to count as necessary on the basis of scientific evidence. Thus, in this opinion scientifically founded clinical guidelines have to decide on the correct use of the term "rationing".[5] The view that rationing involves the limitation of goods regarded as medically necessary is taken by Birnbacher (1999) who states that in the case of "rationing" the standard of delivery (that is the standard of what health care services are societally and politically regarded as important enough to be financed collectively) remains – by definition – below the standard of what is generally considered as medically necessary.

Another standpoint claims that the "medical benefit" – in the German debates: "das medizinisch Sinnvolle" – or "uncontroversial medical benefits" are the adequate reference point. Ubel and Goold (1998) argue that if we are looking for an adequate reference point of limitation we ought to choose the measures which are medically beneficial instead of those that are medically necessary.

A third proposal makes use of the economic terminology of supply and demand. It relies on individual desires as the standard of limitation and hence unambiguously prefers a *subjective standard*. The use of the word "unambiguously" in this context is well grounded because it certainly could be the case that concepts of rationing which favour remaining below medical efficacy *or* necessity as the standard of limitation prove – perhaps after some efforts of reconstruction – to be

---

[5]   Medical necessity is also chosen by Krimmel (2000) as the standard of limitation. The German physician tries to show that in his country not all medically necessary services are paid for by the public health care insurance. Therefore, he states that rationing is taking place already.

concepts that present rationing as remaining below *desired* or *preferred* quantities.Thus, it does not appear devious to define medical efficacy as something that patients who were medically comprehensively informed would desire or prefer. Be that as it may, if we assume that there already exists a gap between supply and demand in public health and that this gap will unavoidably widen, this concept suggests the proposition that medical goods or services are already rationed and that rationing is necessary.[6] The question then is not *if* rationing is (or will be) an empirical fact but what a policy of healthcare rationing should look like.

A subjective gauge for the standard of limitation would be chosen if we – following Breyer (2000) – agreed on a definition according to which a good A is rationed if and only if A is in a publicly financed health care system provided at a fixed price below the market clearing price and A is not offered to the extent that at least one individual wishes to receive at that price.

2.2
Evaluation-related Differences

The search for evaluation-related differences is guided by the question if in a more or less subtle way value judgments on policies of rationing are implied by certain definitions or usages of the term "rationing" belonging to the limitational concept. In the extreme case we may find "persuasive definitions", i.e. definitions that have as their primary function the transfer of an emotive force from the definiens to the word "rationing" – the definiendum – and thence to the policy of rationing itself.[7] Since it appears to be futile within the limitational concept to define the term in a way that a positive value judgment could be identified, the question is: Do definitions of "rationing" which we find in the current debates and which are examples of the limitational concept differ from the effect that on the one hand there are definitions or usages containing neutral expressions, and on the other hand definitions or usages which emphasize the existing negative associations with the help of certain negatively connotated expressions used in their definiens?

The choice of individual desires, medical benefits or medical necessity as standards of limitation does not imply *as such* a rejection of rationing. Even medical necessity can be chosen as the standard of limitation without *per se* making a decision concerning the justifiability of measures of rationing. And the situation does not even change if "medically necessary" means "necessary for the survival of persons".

We seem to confront a different situation if "rationing" is conceived as the withholding of certain services, if the verb "to withhold s.th. from s.o." is used in the sense of the German phrase *"vorenthalten"*. Among the participants of German debates about health care reform the opinion is widespread that rationing means the *Vorenthaltung* of certain medical goods or services. By using this word in the definiens of the definition of "rationing" it is presupposed that rationing neglects either claims that are derived from positive law or morally justified claims. In any case, on further consideration it seems to be strange or even incoherent to speak of

---

[6]   See Butler (1999) who seems to agree with all of these statements.
[7]   For the concept of persuasive definition e.g. Salmon (1973).

"rationing" as "Vorenthaltung" and to regard rationing as a justifiable health care policy.

Apparently there is a semantic difference between "to deny s.th. to s.o." and "to withhold s.th. from s.o." if the latter verb is used in the sense of "vorenthalten". If we say that a person *denies* something to someone and use the expression in the sense of the German noun "Verweigerung" we do not always presuppose that he ignores a claim of another person. Nevertheless, one can express disapproval even at the definition level of health care rationing by using the verb "to deny s.th. to s.o.". According to Kühn (1998, p 66), who is a declared adversary of "healthcare rationing", "rationing" means the "economically, juridically and ethically legitimated denial of medical services – also in the case that they are clinically accepted and their benefits are no matter of controversy."

This definition suggests that rationing is wrong (by using the word "denial") and that people use arguments belonging to different disciplines (such as ethics) in order to justify this wrong policy. Why does the use of the word "denial" seem to strengthen the negative connotations of the term "rationing"? Probably no one will dispute that rationing by denial can occur; the point in question is rather that by defining the term in this way rationing is reduced to an especially harsh kind of limiting health care resources.[8] For example, the possibility seems to be excluded that rationing is accompanied by the consent of patients (as is imaginable when limitations take place by delaying a medical treatment); whereby the negative connotations of the word "rationing" are underlined.

Still more evident is the negative evaluation of health care rationing in the definition presented by Hadorn and Brook (1991), who suggest that the term should "be used to mean societal toleration of inequitable access" to services deemed necessary. Of course, many definitions make use of weaker formulations to characterize the processes that according to them have to be called "health care rationing". The economic definition mentioned above (at the end of the last section) is only one example.

2.3
Differences Concerning the Level of Decision Taking

In addition to the types of differences just mentioned, the usage of the term "rationing" differs with regard to the question whether rationing concerns limitations at the level of budgetary decisions and/or occurs at a lower level at which scarce medical resources have to be allocated to patients. At the one level (the macro level resp. the primary level) scarcity of medical resources is produced, at the other level (the micro level, the secondary level) scarcity already exists as a consequence of budgetary decisions or as a consequence of other policies or circumstances. It is worth noting that at both levels the allocation can be governed by strict and overt rules. An example for such rules at the secondary level are explicit age-limits that determine who gets a scarce transplant.

---

[8]   For different types of rationing see Klein et al. (1996) who describe "rationing by denial" as the "most brutal (and visible) form of rationing" (p 11).

The opinion that the term "rationing" should only be used with regard to a higher level is unambiguously represented by a definition of Mielck and John (1996) that equates rationing with the exclusion of certain "medically efficacious [sinnvollen] and available" services from the catalogue of the public health care insurance [Gesetzliche Krankenversicherung]. Moody (1991) pursues the opposite direction. In an essay about age-based limits in health care he distinguishes between allocation and rationing and proposes to reserve the term "allocation" for decisions made on a higher, collective level while according to his definition the term "rationing" is correctly used only with regard to the individual level of decision making.[9] According to the latter conception that confines the use of the expression "rationing" to the individual level selections of patients for scarce intensive care would be typical examples for rationing. According to the former conception that confines the use of the same expression to a higher level, this could be an "allocation of scarce resources", but certainly not "rationing".

A well-known alternative to these conceptions is to use the terminology of "rationing" with regard to at least two levels – on the one hand the individual level and on the other hand the level at which the resources of certain sectors in public health – for example the number of beds for an intensive care unit – are determined. The labels "microrationing" and "macrorationing" are instruments actually being used to differentiate between the levels.[10] Ubel and Goold (1998) refer explicitly to both levels when they fix the meaning of the term in a broad way.[11]

The following diagram sums up our proposal as to how the alternative concepts of "rationing", that stress the limitational aspect could be classified. It also shows how those authors who are mentioned in the last sections and who define or use the term "health care rationing" in this sense could be classified within our scheme.[12] Where authors do not explicitly want to restrict the use of that term to only one level it is normally assumed that they refer to both levels – the micro level and the

---

[9] Moody defines "rationing" as "a clear and direct limitation of access to an existing scarce good or service at the individual level, when the limit is imposed according to some categorical criteria other than the market." (p 196). On grounds of political feasibility he argues for an age-based allocation scheme (like Medicare) instead of a policy of age-based rationing. See also the very similar definition proposed by the Scandinavians Nilstun and Ohlsson (1995) who want to confine the use of the term "rationing" to "distributional decisions at the individual level involving clear and direct limitation of access to beneficial health care according to some categorial criterion other than the market." (p 81).

[10] See Klein et al. (1996).

[11] They criticize the proposals of some authors to attach the terms "rationing" and "allocation" to different levels of decision making and favor instead an "interpretation of health care rationing that encompasses any explicit or implicit measures that allow people to go without beneficial health care services." (p 209). In contrast, Birnbacher's (1999) statement seems to exhibit an interesting ambiguity because he speaks of "rationing" in terms of the distribution of (elementary) scarce goods such as butter or sugar. It seems to make sense to take account of the distribution of such goods only with regard to the micro level. On the other hand he argues that not all allocational decisions on the micro level as well as on the macro level are rationing decisions. This proposition seems to suggest that rationing is not confined to only one level.

[12] It will hardly be necessary to say that it is not claimed that the names quoted in the cells below amount to a complete enumeration of those proponents who represent the conceptions of rationing in question. Further, it could be the case that there are names that could fill the empty cells.

macro level of decision making. Only if "rationing" is reduced to the denial of goods is it supposed that rationing relates only to the micro level because "to deny s.th. to s.o." obviously means that individuals are turned away.

Table 1. Differences within the concept of rationing as limitation

Levels/ evaluation	Either micro level or macro level		Both levels	
Standards of limitation	Negative	Neutral	Negative	Neutral
Medical efficacy (benefit)	*Micro level:* Kühn	*Micro level:* Nilstun/ Ohlsson *Macro level:* Mielck/John		Ubel/ Goold
Medical necessity			Hadorn/ Brook	Krimmel; Birnbacher
Subjective Standard (desires, preferences)				Breyer
Unspecific		*Micro level:* Moody		Rebscher

2.4
Some Problems of Current Definitions of "Health Care Rationing"

At least some concepts of "health care rationing" are questionable. For example, relying on *medical necessity* or *medical benefit* as standards of limitation is problematic because these expressions are vague. Because of their vagueness definitions that make use of these expressions face problems which – following the sorites paradox discussed by logicians – can be called "sorites problems" (from Greek "sorós" = heap).[13] Certainly there are medical interventions the necessity of which cannot be disputed seriously. An intervention the omission of which would lead to the death of a patient within a few hours is medically necessary beyond question. But on the other hand there are medical measures that do not allow definite answers. For example, the question arises what amount of nursing is "necessary" or "beneficial" for comatose patients. There are constellations of grains of sand allowing no definite answer to the question whether they form a heap. In case of the expressions "medically necessary" or "medically beneficial"

---

[13] In the classical sorites paradox one moves from the true proposition that e.g. a constellation of grains of sand constitutes a heap – and through the further assumption that a heap of sand from which one takes one grain continues to be a heap – to absurd propositions such as the proposition that one single grain of sand is a heap. See Sainsbury (1988).

we are similarily confronted with the difficulty of not always being able to decide whether particular measures belong to their extension.

Choosing medical necessity or medical benefit as standards of limitation suggests that the task of drawing a line between necessary and merely beneficial or between beneficial and futile interventions is delegated to the medical profession. Thereby, the danger emerges that difficult moral judgments are widely perceived as ordinary judgments of medical science and value judgments of dubious value are regarded as judgments of scientific dignity.[14] Moreover, because of the vagueness of the expressions in question it becomes easier for officials, politicians and insurances to belittle momentuous allocational decisions.[15] Thus, it is obvious that the delegation of setting the standard of limitation to the medical profession makes political and societal control of allocational decisions in medicine more complicated.

The most important problem of the definition according to which individual desires or preferences are the standard of limitation (see section 2.1) probably lies in the proviso that there must only be one individual who wants more of a collectively financed service. Because there is probably always someone who wishes more of such goods it is hardly possible on the basis of this definition to distinguish between a purely allocational concept of rationing on the one hand and a limitational concept of rationing on the other hand. However, the definition seems to avoid the problems of the concepts of rationing that refer to medical necessity or medical efficacy and it focuses the attention less on problematic distinctions than on whether particular kinds of limiting health care resources are appropriate.[16]

Let us take a look at reduction of rationing to the *denial* or *withholding* of certain medical goods or services. First, at least definitions equating rationing with the withholding of certain medical goods or services are apparently not appropriate with regard to the allocation of health care services in liberal societies because they suggest that there is no other possibility for individuals to get these services than from collectively financed healthcare. Second, according to the usage of the expression "to withhold s.th. from s.o." in the sense of the German verb "vorenthalten" it is presupposed that there exists a claim to the goods withheld. This claim should be explicitly presented and in doing so it has to be plausibly argued that people should get certain health care services on legal and/or moral grounds. Further explicational efforts also seem to be necessary if one prefers the definition favored by Hadorn/Brook (see above section 2.2), because at least the expression "inequitable distribution" occurring in the definiens is certainly not precise enough. After all, this expression as well as the use of the verbs "to withhold s.th. from s.o." and "to deny

---

[14] This objection is inspired by Ubel and Goold (1998) who argue against Hadorn and Brook that "by equating the withholding of necessary services with rationing, they make it too easy for others to ignore the difficult moral judgments crucial to any determination of necessary benefits." (p 212). Nevertheless, to determine which services are truly beneficial also seems to require difficult value judgments, as Ubel and Goold admit.

[15] As Krimmel (2000) plausibly states, the belittling of serious limitations is fostered by the wide range of interpretations the expression "medical necessity" offers.

[16] See again Ubel and Goold (1998) who plead on similar grounds for a broad definition of "health care rationing".

s.th. to s.o." strengthen the negative connotations of the term "rationing" and for that reason they impede unbiased debates about the future of publicly financed health care.

By restricting rationing *per definitionem* to one *level of decision making*, for example to the individual level, alternative terms have to be chosen for the other level(s). According to Ubel and Goold (1998) the term "health care rationing" suggests in itself "difficult decisions with potentially tragic consequences" (p 210). As these authors plausibly argue the wrong impression can be produced that decisions made on another level are less grave because other terms lack these weighty connotations.

If we favor a limitational concept of rationing the procedure of explication should from my own point of view result in the acceptance of a definition that includes the possibility of rationing on all levels at which allocational decisions in public health are made. Further, the definition should refer to individual desires (or preferences) and to medical standards such as medical necessity or benefit only if they are reduced to individual desires or preferences. Finally, it should contribute to an unbiased debate about the future of publicly financed health care by using neutral expressions in its definiens.

3
References

Birnbacher D (1999) Ethische Probleme der Rationierung im Gesundheitswesen. In: Brudermüller G (Hrsg.) Angewandte Ethik und Medizin. Königshausen & Neumann, Würzburg

Breyer F (2000) Zukunftsperspektiven der Gesundheitssicherung. In: Hauser R (Hrsg.), Zukunft des Sozialstaats. Duncker & Humblot, Berlin

Hadorn DC, Brook RH (1991) The Health Care Resource Allocation Debate. Defining Our Terms. In: JAMA 266, pp 3328–31

Klein R, Day P, Redmayne S (1996) Managing Scarcity. Priority Setting and Rationing in the National Health Service. Open University Press, Buckingham/Bristol

Kliemt H (1998) Gesundheitsversorgung bei Ressourcenknappheit. In: Nagel E, Fuchs C (Hrsg.) Rationalisierung und Rationierung im deutschen Gesundheitswesen. Thieme

Krimmel L (2000) Stiller Abschied vom "medizinisch Notwendigen". In: Deutsches Ärzteblatt 97, A-1052–1053

Kühn H (1998) Rationierende Medizin: Praxis und Ideologie der "Rationierung" in den USA und Großbritannien. In: Kaupen-Haas H, Rothmaler C (Hrsg.) Strategien der Gesundheits-ökonomie, Sozialhygiene und Public Health. Bd. 4, Mabuse, Frankfurt/M.

Mielck A, John J (1996) Kostendämpfung im Gesundheitswesen durch Rationierung – Was spricht dafür und was dagegen? In: Gesundheitswesen (58), pp 1–9

Moody HR (1991) Allocation, Yes; Age-based Rationing, No. In: Binstock RH, Post SG (Hrsg.) Too Old For Health Care? Controversies in Medicine, Law, Economics, and Ethics. The Johns Hopkins University Press, Baltimore/London

Nilstun T, Ohlsson R (1995) Should Health Care be Rationied by Age? In: Scand. J. Soc. Med. (23), pp 81–84

Rebscher H (1998) Rationalisierung und Rationierung im deutschen Gesundheitswesen. In: Nagel E, Fuchs C (Hrsg.) Rationalisierung und Rationierung im deutschen Gesundheitswesen. Thieme

Sainsbury RM (1993) Paradoxes. Cambridge University Press, Cambridge

Salmon WC (1973) Logic. Prentice-Hall (Second Edition), Englewood Cliffs

Siegwart G (1997) Explikation. Ein methodologischer Versuch. In: Löffler W, Runggaldier E
    (Hrsg.) Dialog und System. Otto Muck zum 65. Geburtstag. Academia Verlag, Sankt Augustin

Smith R (1998) Plädoyer für eine offene Rationierungsdebatte. In: Dt Ärztebl 95: A-2453–2458

Ubel PA, Goold SD (1998) 'Rationing' Health Care. Not All Definitions Are Created Equal. In:
    Arch Intern Med 158, pp 209–214

Prioritizing and Rationing

Heiner Raspe

1
Introduction

To begin with, I have to thank the organizers for inviting me to this promising conference. I am especially grateful to Dr. Kliemt for his initial contact. Second, I would like to introduce myself to clarify the background of my considerations: Precisely speaking, there are two backgrounds: one is clinical, the other is sociology. I am now the head of an Institute for Social Medicine within a medical faculty, trying to combine clinical and sociological reasoning in epidemiology and health services research. Finally, I am co-author of a recently published statement of the Central Ethical Commission at our Federal Board of Physicians. It is on "Priorities in Medical Care" within our system of statuatory health insurance. A part of my presentation will deal with this paper and present some of its basic ideas.

Before that however I have to comment on differences between prioritizing and rationing, concepts which are often and erroneously identified with each other. I would like to distinguish the two by their prerequisites, concepts, actors, actions and consequences. Finally I propose some practical steps to promote the debate on priorities in health care in our country.

2
Prioritizing and/or Rationing?

The driving forces behind prioritizing and/or rationing seem to be similar, if not identical. I will not go into details here. However, we are all aware of increasing medical needs, demands and supply (with the problem of supply induced demand) on one hand and the limited financial and infrastructural ressources on the other. This contradiction is painful at least for social systems which meet three criteria:

- being financed by taxes or compulsory contributions,
- committing themselves to keeping their taxes or contributions stable and
- having been subscribing to basic rules of solidarity, social equity and justice.

Increases in need, demand and supply are in themselves determined by nearly uncontrollable processes, such as the demographic transition, the epidemiological transition and the ever accelerating medical progress. New technologies are usually additive to and more expensive than what is presently in use.

In 1997 delegates to a NHS-conference in London wrote to the prior Secreetary of Health that they agreed "that not all health services can be provided to everybody who might benefit from them. This will remain true even with more generous funding, greater efficiency, and lower management costs" (BMJ 1997; 315:147). They proposed, what they called "smart rationing" – which means "thinking about the value of health services not just their costs".

Thus the scene for a debate on rationing is set with rationing defined as systematically withholding medical interventions which are either necessary or potentially benefical and demanded by or at least acceptable for patients.

The use of the word "necessary" in Germany, especially in its social, civil and public law is often vague and inconsistent. In the context of medicine I propose to use it primarily in the strict sense of a "nessecary condition", i.e. an intervention without which a medically desirable effect will not occur. If additionally a patient's life is at risk, clinicians would speak of an "absolute indication" to act. We have to acknowledge however that there are not too many absolute indications in clinical medicine. There aren't too many lethal or severely disabling conditions upon which you must react in due time and with means that have no alternative. It is currently open how severe a disease state and how effective an irreplaceable remedy must be to suggest its "necessity". Most indications in medicine are, as doctors say, "relative": you have time to consider and plan them carefully and there are functional equivalents. Some of those treatments are nevertheless highly effective and – more important – highly useful, others are less so, some are of proven uselessness and some are likely to cause more harm than benefit.

If this is true: what should be the first target of rationing? We all, I am convinced, will agree that rationing should start in the periphery of the less useful interventions and indications. The small range of "the absolutely necessary" should be protected as long as possible.

And if this is true, distinguishing the absolutly necessary from the relatively necessary and the merely useful and the very useful from the less useful interventions becomes unavoidable. And that is what prioritizing is aiming at.

In other words: *Prioritizing is the intellectual and social prerequisite of rationing.* You must not ration in the absence of clear priorities.

There are more differences between the two concepts: they require different actions, actors, and addressees.

– Priorities are to be carefully considered and developed, rationing has to be executed.
– In prioritizing the first step is to examine patients' and residents' needs on the basis of sound empirical evidence. Mainly evidence for the subjects' *ability to benefit* from various diagnostic, preventive, therapeutic etc. interventions. In rationing the first step is to clarify means and readiness among those who carry structural responsibilities.
– Prioritizing requires multiprofessional input, mainly from representatives of clinical and methodological disciplines, including various types of clinicians (physicians, nurses, physios, psychologists, social worker etc.), epidemiologists, biostatisticians, health oeconomists, jurists and ethicists. Rationing requires juridical considerations as well as political negotiations and conclusive decisions.
– After first developments priorities have to be proposed to further professional

and patient groups, and in fact the general public. They are to be discussed openly and within democratically legitimized institutions. Rationing has to be assigned to and finally executed by authoritative albeit democratically legitimized institutions.

– Rationing knows only two extremes, black and white: Prioritizing is aware of a broad range of grey colours.
– Prioritizing prepares and supports not only rationing but rationalization as well.

After all it seems difficult not to separate the developement of priorities from the act of rationing. If rationing in health care is to become our certain fate (as Maynard and Bloor have put it (1998)), then only after a careful consideration of priorities.

3
The Statement of the Central Ethical Commission at the Federal Chamber of Physicians of Germany

This is the main reason why the a.m. Central Ethical Commision (ZEKO) has tried to focus the German discussion first on prioritizing. We are aware of the disappointment of many who already expected us to provide clear cut criteria on what to include in and exclude from a basket of basic health care ("Grundversorgung").

We thought we should not miss the second chance of becoming familiar with the concepts, methods and techniques of evidence-based clinical medicine and evidence-based health care. The *second* chance? We had a first in the early thirties of the last century. It was in 1932 when Paul Martini published the first edition of his "Methodenlehre der Therapeutisch-Klinischen Forschung" ("methods of clinical therapeutical research"). Paul Martini seemed to be one of the world's first clinical epidemiologists (Sackett 1969). Most recently, his life and work found the interest of the international readership of the LANCET (Shelley and Baur 1999). As many other progressive initiatives this was buried and forgotten during the time of the Nazi regime. After the war it never regained its early momentum. We now have to import evidence-based medicine and evidence-based health care from the anglophone world, mainly Canada and the UK – interestingly two countries with a strong tradition as social welfare states.

This reminds us of an essential prerequisite of prioritizing: it requires a community of individuals connected by mutual dependence, responsibility and solidarity. Prioritizing is unnecessary, useless and even inconceivable in both pure market economies and paradise. In either case subjects are driven and ruled by idiosyncratic preferences, not by social priorities. Setting priorities is thus a matter of benevolent paternalism and more or less uncompatible with the notion of patients as sovereign customers. A central element of the concept of priorization is the idea of health care needs. Need has to be distinguished from demand, supply, and actual care. Needs can and must be objectified, at least in part. This idea is easily understood by physicians. We believe in, more than that: we live on the concept of indications. Making indications is a basic medical activity. Indications connect health problems with appropriate remedies. You have already heard of the distinctions between absolut and relative indications.

The activity of making indications is governed by rules based on so called "best available external clinical evidence from systematic research" (Sackett et al. 1996). On this scientific fundament indications produced the famous "condition-treatment pairs" of the Oregon Health Plan, a prioritizing exercise within a Medicaid programme. We can now understand the British definition of need as "what people might benefit from" (Stevens and Raftery 1994). When there is no ability or capacity to benefit *from* health care, then there is no need *for* health care. And this brings us to clinical evaluative research, evidence-based medicine and health technology assessment, since our knowledge of possible benefits and harms of any diagnostic and therapeutic intervention solely depends on prior medical experience, at best collective experience from controlled clinical trials.

If you accept this precondition then it is only a short way to the idea that needs may differ widely in terms of relevance and urgency, depending on the

- status and relevance of the health problem involved,
- the relevance and dignity of the respective therapeutic target,
- the efficacy and effectiveness of the interventions,
- their risks and costs, and
- their acceptability for patients and the public.

Many regard female macro- or micromastia a health problem in itself. Health care systems tend to accept this view and pay for an operative correction only if the condition have been leading to further mechanical or psychological disorder. If not it is, in their view, no relevant health problem and the production of beauty not a dignified therapeutic aim. Comparable examples are infertility treatment or tattoo removing.

On the other hand: not every life-threatening situation does per se imply a need (as defined above). I dare to remind you of the "tragic choices" (Ham and Pickard 1998) that in early 1995 had to be made in one English health authority. Its administration and head physician refused to fund a second bone marrow transplant for Child B (a girl with secondary leucaemia) solely on the ground of trading off a very low chance of survival (estimated below 3 per cent) against very high costs mainly in terms of suffering and side-effects of the intervention. It was said to be a matter of ineffectiveness and inappropriateness of the treatment requested by the child's father and a doctor not primarily involved in the case. The denial survived two court battles.

Nevertheless the girl was transplanted and the costs were covered by a private benefactor. The girl first survived the intervention and died a few months later.

This example shows that even interventions without any alternative (and a bone marrow transplant has no functional equivalent in such a case) have to be prioritized, not to speak of health care interventions which are "only" useful and not necessary in the strict sense of the word. We can identify at last three elements of in a strict sense necessary interventions: the presence of a serious health problem, availability of an effective intervention, and the absence of a convincing alternative. As terms like "serious", "effective" and "convincing" are value-loaden and in need of further clarification the whole definition is far from being precise.

In summary: Need is not a dichotomous category (need vs. no need); but there is always more or less need. Only this fact makes priority setting possible and in itself necessary. To my opinion, it has no alternative. Priority setting hence implies ordinal scaling resulting in hierarchies of interventions or indications. Top ranks are assigned to indispensible low-risk interventions in urgent and otherwise life-threatening situations. Low ranks are assigned to either trivial health problems or to interventions with no proven use or more unfavourable than favourable effects.

The statements show how complex, difficult, and value-loaden it is to develop priorities in health care. The time of simple solutions is definitely over. The Central Ethical Commission proposed to set up a national priorities committee, not to complete a catalogue of undisputable priorities but rather to inform, lead and accompany the national discussion which is to be started and moved forward – with a delay of about ten years compared to other European countries.

4
Finally some Practical Suggestions

The Oregon experiment lead to a single list of more than 700 priorities and posteriorities from all fields of preventive, curative and rehabilitative medicine. It is unlikely that such an experiment will ever be repeated, at least not in communities with 50, 60 or 80 millions of residents. It looks more like a tribal solution.

Instead I propose to try to prioritize – in a first step – indications from single disciplines such as orthopaedic surgery and then in a second step differential indications within an even smaller field of practice such as hip or knee replacement. This would help to get experience in preparing, devolping and discussing priorities.

Let me illustrate the first step: Table 1 shows strata of priorities, each with some paradigmatic conditions from the field of rheumatology. It considers the worst possible outcome without treatment and the best possible outcome under treatment, i.e. the natural vs. clinical course of different types of conditions.

A high priority may be given to an acute fatal disease which can be cured completely, a rather rare event in rheumatological practice. At the bottom there are self healing conditions the recovery from which treatment can but accelerated. Between the two extremes we have different types of conditions some of which may lead to severe and/or lasting disabilities and may be cured or effectively trea-ted or at least alleviated. Though this order may be acceptable or even trivial, many open questions remain:

- what level and quality of evidence do we require,
- from what type of study (confirmatory vs. observtional),
- for what – more or less relevant and valuable – effects,
- for what effect sizes and likelihoods (expressed for instance as relative risk reductions (RRR) and numbers needed to treat (NNT)),
- for what duration,
- what balance between desirable and undesirable effects (numbers needed to harm (NNH)/NNT),
- at what direct, indirect and intangible costs?

Typical answers to any of these questions include words as "high", "socially desirable", "acceptable", "sufficient" etc. – indicating that in any case a judgement

Table 1. Strata of Priorities and some Paradigmatic Indications (Rheumatology)

Worst Likely Outcome if untreated	Best if treated	Example
Premature Death	Cure	Septic Arthritis M. Whipple
	Residue	M. Wegener sp Rheumatoid Arthritis
Death	Palliation	Terminal Care
Severe and/or Lasting Disability	Cure	OA Knee (TNR) - N Gout
	Residue	sn Rheumatoid Arthritis Fragility Fracture Congenital Deformity
	Relief	Fibromyalgia
Minor and/or Transient Disability	Cure Residue	Traumatic Fracture OA Hands Nonspecific Back Pain Fibromyalgia
	Relief	Foot Deformity
Non-disabling Impairment	Relief	OA Hands
Self Healing	Rapid Recovery	Sprains and Strains Reactive Arthritis
Death, Disability	Non-Occurrence	1°, 2°, 3° Prevention (Osteoporosis, Falls)

Open Questions:
- Quality of Evidence for Effectiveness?
- Effect Size? NNT? NNH?
- Direct, indirect, intangible Cost?
- Special Groups: elderly, children, other vulnerable?

is to be made on the grounds of social norms and values. There are further questions: How can the perspective of the general public be taken into account (given our political system of a representative democracy); what about special groups which receive higher or lower than average priorities. In a local survey in Lübeck, any type of service ranked high when beneficial for children and many ranked low when elderly were involved (Westpfahl et al. 2001). And what about prevention? Has it always to be put aside or postponed? Its effects are virtually never directly visible, often delayed for years and with a low chance of occurence. The tacitly invoked "law of rescue" has an interesting analogy to the concept of discounting in health oeconomics (cf. Dialog Ethik 1999).

The proposal for the second step follows a concept which has been developed in New Zealand since 1992, inter alia for total hip and knee replacement. In situations where major joint replacement is to be considered each single patient is assessed by means of a standardised multidimensional score. It covers four principal components: pain, functional activity, movement and deformity and other factors. At worst a patient can reach a score of 100 indicating that he or she is in an untolerable condition and should have an operation as early as possible (Hadorn and Holmes 1997).

This approach reflects an experience that many countries have made: *there are not too many services that can be excluded from coverage once and for all*. Most services confer more or less benefit, depending on the clinical, psychosocial and infrastructural circumstances under which patient *and* provider meet.

Thus general exclusions have to be reconsidered in the light of idiosyncratic situations. And general inclusions have to be targeted on those in greater need according to established indication rules. If distributed too widely the use of a service runs the risk of becoming inappropriate or inadequate. Many studies have shown that the percentage of an inappropriate use of in itself useful and evidence-based interventions easily exceeds 30 per cent, 40 per cent and even 50 per cent.

Concluding remarks:

1. It should have become clear that a review of the best available empirical evidence for benefits and risks of a medical intervention or service does form the heart of priorization.

2. It should have become clear that a second basis (or is it the first and more important?) is to be formed by ethical considerations. The Swedish Parliamentary Priorities Commission (1995) proposed "three principles on which priorities should be based": the principle of human dignity, the principle of need and solidarity and the principle of cost-efficiency (p 103).

   Different criteria will lead to different results. And each set of criteria has both ethical and pragmatic consequences: Ranking high for instance the autonomy of patients and/or clinicians would interfere with the more paternalistic attitude so characteristic for setting priorities in social welfare states. It may additionally lead to a wider and deeper involvement of the public (Mullen and Spurgeon 2000). And it may lead to a comparatively broad range of services which may be left to individual responsibility.

   Emphasizing utilitarian concepts would make it difficult to give high ranks to rare and costly conditions (such as liver transplants) or to patients with an already reduced life span. This is why our commission orientated itself first on the clinical principle of individual need and second on the principle of formal justice which says that equals (equals in respect to their medical need) must be treated equally and unequals unequally.

3. A final point: though the Commission strongly recommended to develop priorities at the level of the whole of our health care system, eventually any priorities have to be accepted and adopted on a regional and finally local basis. Top-down priorities may interfere with already existing priorities or preferences as expressed in daily medical routines, infrastucture and vested interests. And there we have the third basis of priorization: the valid exploration of the existing reality of medical care in a given country, region and organization.

This makes it again clear why priorization is a slow and difficult undertaking which inevitably will cause conflicts. They have to be clarified, discussed and attenuated before open and hard rationing is to be executed.

5
References

Maynard A, Bloor K (1998) Our certain fate: Rationing in health care. Office of Health Economics, London

Martini P (1932) Methodenlehre der therapeutisch-klinischen Forschung. Springer, Berlin

Sackett D (1969) Clinical Epidemiology. Am J Epidemiol 89, pp 125–128

Shelley JH, Baur MP (1999) Paul Martini: the first clinical pharmacologist? Lancet 353, pp 1870–1873

Sackett DL, Rosenberg WMC, Muir Gray JA et al. (1996) Evidence-based medicine: What it is and what it isn't. BMJ 312, pp 71–72

Stevens A, Raftery J (eds) (1994) Health care needs assessment. Redcliff Medical Press, Oxford

Ham C, Pickard S (1998) Tragic choices in health care. King's Fund Publishing, London

Westphal R, Röstermundt A, Raspe H (im Druck) Die Bedeutung ausgewählter präventiver, therapeutischer und rehabilitativer Leistungen im Spiegel eines Bevölkerungssurveys. Gesundheitswesen

Dialog Ethik: Manifest für eine faire Mittelverteilung im Gesundheitswesen. Schweizerische Ärztezeitung 80 (1999) pp 1–9

Hadorn DC, Holmes AC (1997) The New Zealand priority criteria project. Part I: Overview. Brit Med J 314, pp 131–134

The Swedish Parliamentary Priorities Commission: Priorities in Health Care. The Ministry of Health and Social Affairs, Stockholm Offsetcentral (1995)

Mullen P, Spurgeon P (2000) Priority Setting and The Public. Oxon, Radcliffe Medical Press

The Practice of Rationing Health Care in the United Kingdom

David J. Hunter

1
Introduction

The rationing of health care is one of those 'wicked issues' to which there is no easy solution and possibly none at all. In the British National Health Service (NHS) rationing only entered common currency in the early 1990s when the Conservative government introduced its internal market changes. At this point, the process of allocating resources, which had up until then been shrouded in mystery and notions of clinical judgement, became more explicit as a result of the purchaser-provider separation and the emergence of a contract culture between the funders and planners of services on the one hand and those providing them on the other.

However, rationing as a phenomenon has always existed – it is the terminology that has changed. Until the 1991 NHS reforms, terms like 'priority-setting' and 'making choices' were in common usage. As one commentator has put it: 'priority-setting' is viewed as a term which makes rationing 'sound a little less grim, and a little more scientific, than in fact it is' (Loughlin 1996, p 146).

This article reviews the rationing debate in the UK, drawing on the experience of other countries where appropriate, and examines the arguments in favour of explicit and implicit rationing respectively. It concludes by arguing that rationing is an unwinnable dilemma of public policy. There are no solutions to some problems and we should not allow the rational-scientific bias that underlies much of the discourse in public policy to suggest otherwise. Hence the attractions of an approach based on 'muddling through elegantly' (Hunter 1993, Hunter 1998). While we can improve the muddling, it is politically naive to think that there is a winning formula waiting to be discovered which will serve as a way of resolving the rationing dilemma once and for all.

2
The Rationing Dilemma

The problem of allocating scarce resources in health care has always existed, and not just in Britain. It is a truism to assert that setting priorities and choosing where and how to invest resources are unavoidable political and management tasks. However, not all commentators accept that rationing is inevitable or that we should embrace it, however reluctantly. A former United States health secretary of state has said: 'rationing is not a solution to the problems we face, it is a capitulation of de-spair' (Califano 1992). And Loughlin (1996, p 147) takes to task health economists and others who profess to have solutions to problems like establishing priorities and whose 'toxic effect' is to obscure 'the monstrous irrationality and barbarity' of modern society. He continues: 'the assumption that there must be a defensible, determinate answer to questions about who should be allowed to suffer and die, is false' (p 155).

The dilemma faced by the rational rationers, or those who insist upon the purification qualities of making hard choices, is that their position is simplistic and politically naive. At a normative level, they may be right. It would be intrinsically desirable to have a system of resource allocation bounded by clear rules and procedures. But no such system can be sensitive to the myriad complexities surrounding the care of people with multiple needs and varying social circumstances. Moreover, we tend to overstate the miracle of modern medicine. As the United States Surgeon-General has said, the best estimates are that health services affect about 10 per cent of the usual indices for measuring health: infant mortality, absences through sickness, and adult mortality. The remaining 90 per cent are determined by factors over which health services have little or no control: individual lifestyle, social conditions, and the physical environment. In the words of one policy analyst: 'no one is saying that medicine is good for nothing, only that it is not good for everything' (Wildavsky 1979).

Whatever other arguments may be mobilised concerning the defeatism to which a focus on rationing can give rise, the prevailing orthodoxy in Britain, as elsewhere, is that rationing is both inevitable and should be made more explicit.

3
Defining Terms

Rationing can be defined in a variety of ways. In its evidence to the House of Commons Health Committee (1995), the Association of Community Health Councils for England and Wales identified three distinct forms of rationing:

- withdrawal of the NHS from a particular type of service or treatment (e.g. 'cosmetic' operations, treatment of infertility, tattoo removal, long-term care of the elderly);
- explicit and regular attempts to define how much of which services should be provided and moving resources between services;
- restricting access to a service by reference to the characteristics of prospective patients, e.g. their age, personal lifestyle (whether they smoke, take drugs, are heavy drinkers and so on).

Briefly examining each of these in turn, rationing in the NHS can and does occur commonly through a range of devices such as deterrence, delay, deflection, dilution and denial (Harrison and Hunter 1994, pp 25–30). As Aaron and Schwartz found in their comparative study of rationing in the US and Britain, 'few of the criteria for rejection are explicitly stated. Age, for example, is not officially identified as an obstacle to treatment' (Aaron and Schwartz 1984, p 37). Yet there is very clear evidence that age is a major factor in determining whether treatment is sanctioned or denied (Grimley Evans 1993). However, it is not clear whether rationing is itself a cause of elderly people being denied treatment from which they could benefit or whether it is a symptomatic reflection of deep-seated ageist attitudes within society which are in turn reflected in the treatment decisions made by professionals. In a society plagued by images of 'a rising tide' of elderly people and by the 'burden of ageing' it is hardly surprising that negative stereotypes prevail. Positive views of ageing would be unlikely to be reflected in rationing decisions currently based on age.

Given the inevitability of exercising professional judgement in decisions about who to treat and how, it is almost impossible to trace the motivation underlying the decision. What may be denied a patient on the grounds that they would not benefit from the treatment may in fact be inextricably bound up with moral factors whereby a patient is seen as less deserving and as getting their 'just deserts'. While doctors may be forbidden to allow moral judgements to enter into their decision-making, it may in practice be difficult to disentangle these from clinical judgements. In sum, the content of medical work is a complex mix of clinical factors, effectiveness of resource use and policing lifestyle (Hughes and Griffiths 1996).

While those concerned about the value-laden nature of much professional decision-making advocate explicit rationing as a way of exposing and holding to account the making of moral judgements, there is no a priori reason to believe that explicit rationing would in fact be any more rational. As Hughes and Griffiths state: 'It is perfectly possible for doctors to act according to their perceptions of deservingness, while accounting for their actions in terms of medical benefit'. But in situations of tight resource constraints, making treatment decisions on clinical grounds alone may not be sufficient. Inevitably, therefore, moral factors come into play.

In the NHS, priority-setting has largely been left to health authorities and, in future, it will progressively become the responsibility of primary care groups and trusts (at least in England; different arrangements exist in Wales, Scotland and Northern Ireland). Many health authorities have drawn up lists of procedures they will either not fund at all or only in exceptional circumstances. Most of the exclusions relate to lifestyle treatments that cannot be said to result in major discomfort of a life or death nature. For the most part, too, these exclusions do not release significant savings although the resources made available in this way might be more effectively deployed elsewhere.

Most recent discussion of rationing in the British NHS has been about whether or not it should become more explicit. This is linked to the issue of the level at which rationing should be conducted – national, local, or at the doctor-patient level. In a *national* health system, should it be central government which takes responsibility for what are essentially political decisions about the areas of care and treatment the NHS should cover and exclude? Or is it reasonable to leave such decisions to the local level where there is more knowledge about needs and about the population's characteristics? If the local level is allowed to decide then the likelihood must be that there will be local variations. Why else allow local choice? But the problem then is one of what has been termed 'postcode prescribing', a form of rationing based on where a person happens to live rather than on their need for health care.

4
A National or Local Approach to Rationing?

For many years the British Medical Association and various other health service organisations have been calling on central government to take the lead on rationing and to make explicit decisions instead of looking to health authorities and doctors to take them. Indeed, Richard Smith, editor of the *British Medical Journal*, went so far as to accuse government of a 'failure of leadership' with the result that 'Britain has not had the broad, deep, informed, and prolonged debate on rationing that is needed' (Smith 1995: 686). Britain is accused of lagging behind countries like The Netherlands, Sweden and New Zealand all of which have grasped the nettle of explicit rationing, albeit with varying degrees of success (Hunter 1998).

International experience demonstrates that there exist several approaches to tackling rationing, ranging from prescribed lists of treatment to be included in a publicly funded system of health care, through wide-ranging ethical discussions to establish criteria governing resource use, to agreeing broad principles as the basis of a coherent policy framework (Coulter and Ham (eds), 2000). There is no consensus on the best way forward and all British governments over the years have resisted attempts either to define a set of core services, to rank treatments, or to lead a public debate on the issue other than to reassert the founding principles of the NHS as a universal facility accessible to all in need of care and to reaffirm its view that it is for local health authorities not to ration care or deny effective treatments but to establish priorities informed by public opinion.

An exception to this position has been the introduction into the NHS of the drug Viagra manufactured by Pfizer. For the first time, the arrival of a new drug on the market triggered an intervention by the Secretary of State for Health in order to restrict the circumstances under which it could be prescribed on the NHS. But the case illustrates all the pitfalls of Ministers taking a lead on rationing and is unlikely to be repeated. Moreover, Viagra is not concerned with a life-threatening condition and for a Minister to become directly involved in a life and death matter would be extremely unlikely. As Klein once wrote, governments generally seek to diffuse blame and centralise credit (Klein 1995). But the Viagra example does demonstrate what can happen when governments seek to determine nationally what treatment options should be available and for whom. Having been urged to develop a national policy by clinicians, various NHS organisations and assorted academics the Secretary of State did so in respect of Viagra publishing a list of criteria governing its use on the NHS.

The pronouncement triggered an immediate backlash on the grounds that the list excluded all kinds of deserving medical conditions and that doctors on the frontline were best placed to make such decisions since they knew their patients best. That, after all, is the whole point of professional judgement. As a result of the furore, the government extended its list of inclusions and inserted an escape clause which allowed doctors a certain degree of freedom to prescribe the drug in exceptional circumstances. But there remains criticism of the process and the outcome. Supporters of the government's stance claim that the Minister was absolutely right to react in the way he did even if the resulting decision was defective. But is this not precisely the point? From *somebody's* perspective the outcome will probably always be defective. If the political fallout becomes damaging then it is unlikely that governments will wish to be so explicit in future in quite such a 'hands on' way.

The next best option is to set up a national body to take rationing decisions on behalf of the government but to present them up as evidence-based decisions underpinned by robust science and research evidence. The NHS Research & Development strategy, introduced in 1991, and the ensuing evidence-based medicine (EBM) movement have been attempts to do precisely this and they have not been without some success although there is a risk of raising unrealistic expectations concerning the existence and robustness of an evidence base in respect of all treatments.

In April 1999, the National Institute for Clinical Excellence (NICE) in England and Wales was established (Scotland is pursuing a similar approach with its own machinery). It has produced a steady stream of clinical guidelines and protocols on what works and what does not work. NICE is concerned not just with establishing what is clinically effective but also what is cost-effective. Its Chairman, however, has stated that NICE will not be involved in making rationing decisions. Clinicians will not be compelled to act on the evidence although they will be held accountable for their decisions and be required to give good reasons for not following the appraisals and guidelines produced by NICE.

To ensure that good progress is being made and to assist health authorities, trusts and primary care organisations in changing their practice and behaviour another new national agency for England and Wales, the Commission for Health Improvement (CHI), was set up towards the end of 1999. It provides support and ultimately sanctions if change in management and/or clinical practice is not forthcoming. It is the closest the NHS has come to having its own independent inspectorate although the term is avoided as it tends to produce a negative reaction among clinicians. However, the government is impatient to see evidence of real change in clinical practice and will not hesitate to introduce tougher measures if required. The dilemma remains, however, that in order to secure change the support and compliance of clinicians is needed.

It is far too early to judge how successful NICE and CHI will be but the government regards them as being of critical importance in respect of the rationing issue. Ministers stress that the NHS cannot be expected to provide interventions that are known to be ineffective or where evidence of their efficacy is lacking. But even where relevant studies exist, their application locally may remain problematic. So while NICE may improve the availability, accessibility and dissemination of data, it will be up to CHI to work with health service organisations to encourage their uptake where there is a persistent failure for whatever reason to do so. Through these means, Ministers hope that the lottery of so-called 'post-code rationing' will cease and that a uniform level of provision will exist across the country regardless of where a patient happens to live. The price to pay for this degree of standardisation is greater centralised decision-making and less scope for local variation, and clinical discretion and priority-setting. However, it is hard to see how NICE and CHI will altogether end such practices since it is in the nature of health care and medicine that decisions must reflect individual circumstances which are far from uniform.

NICE will appraise both new and existing technologies covering pharmaceutic-als, medical devices, diagnostic technologies, procedures and health promotion, and will develop and publish clinical guidelines on the basis of its cost-effectiveness analyses. The guidelines will also be available to the public in the hope that patients can establish reasonable expectations and temper unreasonable demands. The evidence base in respect of drug therapies is better than that in the other categories, especially health promotion, although it is unlikely NICE will invest a great deal of its scarce resources on this topic. NICE's recommendations fall into one of three categories: that a treatment or procedure be recommended for routine use in the NHS; that it be recommended for use only in clinical trials; that it not be recommended for routine use. A clinical audit system will accompany each guideline to monitor adherence to NICE's recommendations. Early evidence sug-gests that health authorities often ignore NICE's advice.

Rather less is known about CHI and how it will operate although its director insists that it will adopt a developmental approach in preference to a punitive one. It is charged with the task of offering an independent guarantee that local systems to monitor, assure and improve clinical quality are in place. It will visit all NHS organisations within four years through a system of rolling reviews. Its work pro-gramme is dependent upon a number of successful secondments from the NHS in order to undertake an extensive visiting programme. The work of CHI will comple-ment arrangements for clinical governance. It will offer targeted support and be able to intervene by invitation/request and make recommendations to the Secretary of State for Health.

Both NICE and CHI allow Ministers to be kept at arm's length from making decisions about what treatments work and do not work. The Viagra case illustrates how difficult it is for Ministers to win in such cases even with the weight of public opinion on their side.

The government regards EBM, and a focus on cost-effectiveness in respect of new and existing treatments and interventions, as representing the best way forward. It amounts to a technocratic solution, or fix, to what is essentially a political and social problem or public policy puzzle. Estimates about the amount of resources squandered on ineffective interventions vary. The first NHS R&D Director, Sir Michael Peckham, estimated that at least £1 billion could be released by terminating ineffective procedures. But commentators, like David Eddy, maintain that even eliminating waste, itself very difficult to do, will not obviate the need to ration care (Eddy 1994). At most, it will buy time but that assumes that the evidence base is sufficiently robust and that clinicians will act on the evidence and modify their practice. All the available evidence suggests that even if where is progress it takes a long time to secure. In the meantime pressures on NHS resources intensify.

Responding to these, the Rationing Agenda Group, led by the *British Medical Journal* and King's Fund, have proposed an approach which seeks to be more open and explicit about the principles governing rationing decisions (New and Le Grand 1996). They suggest three basic characteristics that make some kinds of health care special: unpredictability of the need for that care; information imbalance between doctors and patients; and what might be termed the fundamental importance of the care concerned in allowing people to realise their life goals. The application of these principles (none of which would be sufficient on its own) might help in deciding what should be in the NHS and what should lie outside it.

Some interventions are rather obvious and are already the subject of exclusions in some health authorities (as noted above). Within their schema, New and Le Grand argue that cosmetic surgery to enhance physical attractiveness is not of fundamental importance and should not therefore be provided under the NHS. Other treatments and services are less obvious, such as residential care, which can be predicted. It should not therefore be available free under the NHS. But adult dental care and IVF should be available because both are unpredictable. Where New and Le Grand draw the line over being explicit and laying down fairly strict rules is over who should receive treatment and how much they should get. Pragmatism, they believe, should prevail here which means leaving such decisions to clinicians. What a national framework would achieve is an end to the present lottery whereby place of residence can determine whether or not we have a chance of fertility treatments, continuing care, dentistry or whatever.

A difficulty with New and Le Grand's approach, beguiling though it is in its apparent simplicity and reasonableness, is how the characteristic of 'fundamental importance' is to be defined (Klein 1997). An illustration of the dilemma is provided by *in vitro* fertilisation (IVF). Whereas New and Le Grand assert its fundamental importance – 'is not the inability to have a child of fundamental importance?' – the Dunning Committee in The Netherlands which examined the whole issue of making choices in health care excluded IVF from the basic package on the grounds that 'from a community-oriented approach, the answer to the question of necessity would most probably be no' (Ministry of Welfare, Health and Cultural Affairs 1992, p 87).

This sharp divergence of view is the nub of the issue. When there exist multiple interpretations of what constitutes necessity or care of fundamental importance then it renders the whole selection criterion 'vacuous' since it 'provides no guidance on how conflicting interpretations can be resolved' (Klein 1997, p 507). Moreover, for all their efforts to confront 'hard choices' in a hard-nosed fashion, New and Le Grand resort to an 'escape clause' and acknowledge the need for judgement since the three criteria of unpredictability, information imbalance, and fundamental importance are not able 'to specify action so precisely that the need for further thought and judgement is unnecessary' (New and Le Grand 1996, p 52). Individual cases will then need to be assessed so there can be no blanket exclusions. At the end of the day, it would seem, there is no effective substitute for clinical judgement and local discretion albeit within a broad set of principles governing action. But do these not already exist in terms of the NHS's founding principles and core values as laid down in legislation and endorsed by successive governments in white papers and numerous policy statements?

5
Engaging the Public Voice

To resolve the rationing conundrum from another standpoint, which would also have the virtue of tackling what amounts to a significant 'democratic deficit' in the way the NHS is run, policy-makers have resorted to asserting the rights of the public to be actively involved in decisions about who to treat and about what the NHS should cover. Such a participative approach is now common across the public policy landscape, notably in education and in local government.

A dilemma is that members of the public occupy different roles at different times throughout their lives. They can be patients, carers, users of services, taxpayers and citizens. Their views are likely to differ, and certainly be influenced, by the particular role, or roles, they are playing at a particular point in time. Advocates of explicit rationing vary in the extent to which they believe users of services as opposed to citizens should be involved in decisions about resources and who should receive them. So far, efforts to involve the public in making choices about health care have had only limited success. As Moore (1996, p 15) explains:

> Nationally, 'public debate' ends up as media debate, when issues are inevitably treated in a simplistic way. Locally, purchasers have sometimes met with apathy when attempting to debate general principles, while moves to restrict or close services typically prompt vocal opposition.

There are other problems, too. For example, Moore again:

> Asking the general public to weigh up the merits of different demands can produce results which conflict with public health principles. People frequently rank glamorous, high techno-logy services, such as liver transplants, above far more effective and cost effective inter-ventions, like child immunisation and family planning.

Rather than seeking to involve the public at a strategic macro or meso (i.e. local) level in making trade-offs about which sectors or care groups should receive a higher priority, when information and understanding are absent, a better way of involving the public may be at a micro level, i.e. on a one-to-one basis through a more equal partnership with doctors in making decisions about individual treatment (Hunter 1993; Moore 1996). Such an approach is central to effective implicit rationing as articulated through the notion of 'muddling through elegantly'.

This is not to suggest that all attempts at public involvement at a higher level are fatally flawed. To tackle the 'democratic deficit' perceived to exist, there have been numerous experiments with, *inter alia*, health panels, focus groups, citizens' juries (Cooper et al. 1995, Richardson 1997, Lenaghan 1997). Citizens' juries have received a great deal of attention in the United Kingdom and build on earlier models developed in Germany and the United States. The concept draws on the jury system in the courts, arguably the most participative institution in the British state.

The principle uniting all models of citizens' juries is that ordinary citizens, without vested interests or expertise, are able to make sound political decisions if they have enough information and time to consider the issue at stake. Citizens' juries attempt to overcome the passivity which representative government gener-ally assumes and to encourage active citizenship through creative participation. They are not intended to make binding decisions but to consider proposals and make comments and recommendations. It has been suggested that citizens' juries should not be seen in isolation but as one of several innovations, such as delibera-tive opinion polls, mediation groups, referenda and electronic town meetings, designed to strengthen democracy (Stewart et al. 1994). A number of pilot juries have met and been evaluated in the United Kingdom. Many valuable lessons can be learned from these pilot schemes. A key one, apart from the high cost of each jury (in the region of £ 25,000) is that public enthusiasm for juries is tempered by deep cynicism about the possibility of them making a difference. After all, health authorities are not required to take their views into account or even to offer feed-back on how the jury's views have been treated.

Richardson, in her evaluation of the Somerset health panels, concluded that, contrary to the doubts of some analysts, ordinary people are not only willing to take part in rationing discussions but are also capable of exploring complex issues and funding priorities with some sensitivity (Richardson 1997). She asserts that the public can overcome the information asymmetry problem and learn about NHS budget limitations and weigh issues on their merits as well as reflect on the wider implications of their arguments. Richardson believes the results of the Somerset initiative to be sufficiently encouraging to warrant their testing through further such consultation exercises.

6
From Implicit to Explicit Rationing and Back Again?

It appears from reviewing the debate and the reality in Britain, and taking account of developments elsewhere in Europe and beyond, that when all the various initiatives and commission reports on rationing are studied devising acceptable and agreed criteria for rationing is 'a peculiarly intractable endeavour, where practice lags behind rhetoric' (Klein, Day and Redmayne 1996, p 118). Even in New Zea-land, often held up as an example of a country which has done more than any other to involve the public at a macro level in rationing decisions, there is a lack of hard evidence as distinct from speculation as to how effective these efforts have been (Ham and Coulter 2000). There is no generally acceptable technical fix, such as quality adjusted life years (QALYs), for resolving the dilemma posed by finite resources. Nor is there a universal prescription which can be applied. It is not surprising, therefore, for the World Health Organisation (WHO) to conclude its review of health care reform issues in Europe by stating that despite various initiatives to examine priority-setting on a more systematic and explicit basis, 'overall, there has not been any substantial reductions in the coverage or package of benefits offered by [countries'] statutory systems' (WHO 1996, p 106).

If, in keeping with the spirit of the times, rationing is to be explicit and underpinned by a set of publicly agreed principles, then there are a number of variations on this particular theme. At one end of the spectrum there is the option of specifying very tight criteria governing services to be included (and conversely excluded). This is the core service, or restricted menu, or limited list approach. It is sometimes known as the guaranteed entitlement to health care and has, in most countries, been found wanting. New Zealand, where a core service approach was attempted, quickly came to the view that such an approach could not be made to work or be made politically acceptable.

At the other extreme is what may be termed the ethically sound approach. This approach does not seek to exclude any particular service or treatment but rather to establish an agreed public framework of ethics or principles to guide, and not prescribe, decision-making over who should and should not receive treatment. Sweden is perhaps the best example of this approach but it is dismissed by the hard men (for it is men) of rationing who favour hard choices and regard the Swedish 'ethical platform' as vague, insufficiently precise to operationalise and ducking the difficult choices that must be made.

In between these extremes are various approaches, notably the Dutch one, which seeks to combine elements of both approaches: the soft approach to defining and gaining public acceptance for a set of principles to assist in the making of choices, and the hard approach involving the making of specific decisions about who should get treatment (and by definition, if resources are limited, who should be denied it).

Another middle way, and one adopted in Britain, is to firm-up on the evidence base and to refuse to talk of rationing but, instead, use the language of disinvestment in procedures known to be ineffective thereby releasing resources for allocation elsewhere. As long as ineffective procedures are being provided, it is wrong, or at least premature, to talk of rationing. As the Anti-Rationing Group asserts, there is a prior need to terminate ineffective medical interventions (Roberts et al. 1995).

Explicit rationing sounds fine in theory – who in an ideal world could possibly be against an open transparent system of arriving at decisions? But the world is not ideal. It is messy, turbulent, ambivalent and full of paradox. We should not seek to deny or eliminate such aspects but to manage them better. Explicit rationing is not without pitfalls. Five merit brief comment and all are evident in the debate in Britain about rationing health care.

6.1
Whose Voice?

Whose voice is being articulated when public opinion is sought on establishing priorities in health care? Is it the articulate middle class? The 'worried well'? Attempts to engage the public carry the danger of a low priority being attached to the needs of people with a mental illness, a mental handicap, a physical disability, those who are old, and those who are poor and inarticulate. Who will act as advocates on their behalf? Participation is inherently inegalitarian. How far it can and should be relied on in rationing decisions are crucial questions. Even those who favour greater public participation warn that 'it can advantage the already privileged through their ability to manipulate the information process and can sacrifice the common good to sectional interpretations of it' (Doyal and Gough 1991). Of course, it is not impossible to access all sections of a community but the expense and time involved in doing so may act as effective deterrents allowing the more assertive elements of public opinion to hold sway. Implicit rationing is often criticised for sanctioning an inequitable system where 'knowledgeable, sophisticated, and aggressive patients are more able to have their needs satisfied than docile patients' (Mechanic 1995, p 1657). But explicit rationing is also susceptible to a similar bias.

6.2
Quality of Decision-Making

Could explicit decision-making lead to more incremental and conservative decisions at the risk of preventing the development of innovative or different patterns of delivery? Is it possible that reallocating resources from, say, acute to community and primary care or long-term care, difficult though this has been to achieve in the past, could become even more difficult when processes which have been largely implicit become explicit? Merely by increasing the visibility of a decision process, and allowing many more individuals and groups access to it, the potential for conflict among key groups of decision-makers is likely to increase (Mechanic 1995). As Klein (1992, p 5) argues:

> the greater the visibility of rationing in the sense of prioritisation, the more difficult it may become to steer resources towards the most vulnerable ... groups. Lack of visibility may be a necessary condition for the political paternalism required to overcome both consumer and producer lobbies.

6.3
Power of Numbers

As the debate over QALYs and other such techniques has revealed, numbers can have a curiously mesmerising effect on managers and others required to produce, and rely on, them. Often, unfounded assumptions of certainty and precision seem to underpin the very hardness of numbers. But such numbers are an abstraction. They are not an observation of real life: they are generated and produced by a specific set of technical procedures which may be more or less comprehensible to the average manager or non-executive director. It becomes all too easy to forget the value base of numbers and to attach a degree of certainty and precision to them that may be quite unfounded or unwarranted (Carr-Hill 1989). Whatever their value, such techniques should not supplant other, softer qualitative measures or indicators of quality.

6.4
Underfunding is the Issue

Explicit rationing carries the danger that attention is diverted from the real cause of the problem – lack of resources – to its symptoms. A restricted list or core service approach to health care services could lead policy-makers to believe that there is some finite level of health care and level of resources that are appropriate.

6.5
When does covert become overt and vice versa?

The assumption that by being explicit and transparent there is no scope for manipulation and inequitable behaviour is simply naive. Explicit rules are by no means inviolable. As Mechanic concludes, 'the rich and powerful if sufficiently motivated will always find ways to circumvent explicit criteria' (Mechanic 1995, p 1658).

These observations are not intended to imply an uncritical defence of the status quo which suffers from an excess of medical paternalism that is far from satisfactory. But if advocates of an explicit approach believe human behaviour under an implicit approach to be flawed then where is the evidence for believing that it should somehow be different under an explicit system? Zimmern (1996), for example, cautions against being too uncritical about the advantages of transparent and explicit decision-making. Strengthening the rights and autonomy of the individual might be at the expense of the welfare of the collective. Whether or not this is an acceptable price to pay should at least be debated.

7
'Muddling through elegantly'

If overt rationing is a minefield strewn with major problems which could well prove to be as, if not more, intractable than those it seeks to address – a 'wicked issue' as it was described at the outset – then why not consider a rather more subtle and incremental approach which acknowledges the complexities of actual priority-setting? Such an approach has been termed 'muddling through elegantly' (Hunter 1993, 1998).

Muddling through elegantly does not entail a conservative defence of the status quo. Rather, it acknowledges that improvements are necessary in how decisions about priorities are made, especially at a micro level where doctors and patients interact, but that these adjustments can be made within current arrangements backed by a system of procedural rights designed to ensure that the exercise of discretion in decision-making is undertaken fairly thereby ensuring that the principles of equity and equal treatment are upheld (Bynoe 1996, Coote and Hunter 1996).

Procedural rights are based on the principle of fair treatment (in the non-clinical sense). A set of procedural rights in health care might include: a right to be heard, a right to consistency in decision-making, a right to relevance in decision-making, a right to unbiased decisions, a right to reasons, a right to review. Procedural rights are different from substantive rights in that they are not about entitlement to substantive services but about entitlement to fair procedures in the way decisions are reached.

There is no mileage in a wholesale switch to a nationally determined and led system of explicit rationing that is itself unproven. Nobody denies that rationing gives rise to complex moral dilemmas. But to face them explicitly in the manner proposed by the rational rationers may just be too difficult for society to con-template. In support of this position, Gillon (1994, p XXVII) writes:

> Until there is far greater social agreement and indeed understanding of these exceedingly complex issues, I believe that it is morally safer to seek gradual improvement in our current methods of trying to reconcile the competing moral concerns – to seek ways of 'muddling through elegantly' as Hunter advocates, rather than to be seduced by systems that seek to convert these essentially moral choices into apparently scientific numerical methods and formulae.

8
Conclusion

This short discourse on the experience of rationing health care in Britain has sought to counsel against adopting a system of explicit rationing that is not without its own particular flaws and weaknesses. Rationing is a wicked issue. As Stewart defines them, wicked issues are 'deeply intractable' and 'imperfectly understood and to which solutions are not clear' (Stewart 1998, p 19). Health economists' techniques may be tempting in their attempt at precision and simplicity but they reduce the complexity and messiness of real-life policy puzzles and decisions in ways that are ultimately self-defeating.

We should resist abandoning an admittedly imperfect though still workable irrationality in favour of a spurious and possibly risky rationality for the reasons set out above. The goal should be to *satisfice* rather than to optimise. As Mechanic (1995, p 1659) argues, 'interest in making rationing explicit arises from the illusion that optimisation is possible'. Because there is no realistic alternative to *satisficing*, whether from a practical, political or moral standpoint, a strategy of muddling through elegantly may hold particular appeal grounded as it is in pragmatic sensibility backed by a set of procedural rights governing the way individuals are treated and informed about decisions affecting them.

9
References

Aaron, HJ, Schwartz WB (1984) The painful prescription: rationing hospital care. The Brookings Institution, Washington

British Medical Journal (1995) Rationing revisited: a discussion paper. Health Policy and Economic Research Unit Discussion Paper No. 4. BMA, London

Bynoe I (1996) Beyond the citizen's charter. Institute for Public Policy Research, London

Califano JA (1992) Rationing health care – the unnecessary solution. University of Pennsylvania Law Review, 140, pp 1525–38

Carr-Hill RA (1989) Assumptions of the QALY procedure. Social Science and Medicine, 28, pp 469–77

Cooper L, Coote A, Davies A, Jackson C (1995) Voices off: tackling the democratic deficit, Institute for Public Policy Research, London

Coote A, Hunter DJ (1996) New agenda for health. Institute for Public Policy Research, London

Coulter A, Ham C (eds) (2000) The global challenge of health care rationing. Open University Press, Buckingham

Doyal L, Gough I (1991) A theory of human need. Macmillan, London

Eddy D (1994) Health systems reform: will controlling costs require rationing services? Journal of American Medical Association, 272, pp 324–8

Gillon R (1994) Introduction. In: Principles of health care ethics (ed. R Gillon). Wiley & Sons, Chichester

Grimley Evans J (1993) Summary. In: Grimley Evans J, Goldacre MJ, Hodkinson HM, Lamb S, Savory M. Health and function in the third age. Papers prepared for the Carnegie Inquiry into the Third Age. Nuffield Provincial Hospitals Trust, London

Ham C, Coulter A (2000) Conclusion: where are we now? In: Coulter A, Ham C (eds) The global challenge of health care rationing. Open University Press, Buckingham

Harrison S, Hunter DJ (1994) Rationing health care. Institute for Public Policy Research, London

House of Commons Health Committee (1995) Priority-setting in the NHS: purchasing. First report, session 1994–95, volume II, minutes of evidence and appendices, HC 134-II. HMSO, London

Hughes D, Griffiths L (1996) "But if you look at the coronary anatomy …": risk and rationing in cardiac surgery, Sociology of Health and Illness 18, pp 172–97

Hunter DJ (1993) Rationing dilemmas in health care. Research paper number 8. National Association of Health Authorities and Trusts, Birmingham

Hunter DJ (1998) Desperately seeking solutions: rationing health care. Longman, Harlow

Klein R (1992) Dilemmas and decisions. Health Management Quarterly, xiv, pp 2–5

Klein R (1995) The new politics of the NHS. 3rd edition. Longman, Harlow

Klein R (1997) Defining a package of healthcare services the NHS is responsible for: the case against. British Medical Journal, 314, pp 506–9

Klein R, Day P, Redmayne S (1996) Managing scarcity: priority-setting and rationing in the NHS. Open University Press, Buckingham

Lenaghan J (1997) Citizens juries: towards best practice, British Journal of Health Care Management 3, pp 20–22

Loughlin M (1996) Rationing, barbarity and the economist's perspective. Health Care Analysis, 4, pp 146–56

Mechanic D (1995) Dilemmas in rationing health care services: the case for implicit rationing. British Medical Journal, 310, pp 1655–9

Ministry of Welfare, Health and Cultural Affairs (1992) Choices in health care. A report by the Government Committee on Choices in Health Care, The Netherlands. Ministry of Welfare, Health and Cultural Affairs, Rijswijk

Moore W (1996) Hard choices: priority-setting in the NHS. National Association for Health Authorities and Trusts, Birmingham

New B, Le Grand J (1996) Rationing in the NHS: principles and pragmatism. King's Fund, London

Richardson A (1997) Determining priorities for purchasers: the public response to rationing within the NHS, Journal of Management in Medicine 11, pp 222–232

Roberts C, Crosby D, Dunn R, Evans K, Grundy P, Hopkins R, Jones JH, Lewis P, Vetter N, Walker P (1995) Rationing is a desperate measure. Health Service Journal, 105, p 15

Smith R (1995) Editorial: rationing: the debate we have to have. British Medical Journal, 310, p 686

Stewart J (1998) Advance or retreat from the traditions of public administration to the new public management and beyond. Public Policy and Administration, 13, pp 12–27

Stewart J, Kendall E, Coote A (1994) Citizens' juries. Institute for Public Policy Research, London

Wildavsky A (1979) The art and craft of policy analysis. Macmillan, London

World Health Organisation (1996) European health care reform: analysis of current strategies. WHO Regional Office for Europe, Copenhagen

Zimmern R (1996) Beyond effectiveness: the appropriateness of clinical care – what needs to happen now. Transcript of a speech to the National Medical Directors and Directors of Public Health Meeting, November

Comment on Professor David Hunter's Talk

Bettina Schöne-Seifert

Professor Hunter has presented his expert endeavour of "reviewing the debate and reality in Britain" (p 35) with regard to medical rationing. Hence, we have been provided with three different levels of data or theses to think about:

1. the level of *de facto* decision-making upon the provision and non-provision of potentially benefitting care to patients;
2. the level of British reflection thereupon – be it by politicians, by the public, or by academic experts of various backgrounds;
3. the level of Professor Hunter's own theoretical inferences not the least from those very realities and debates.

Let us have a brief look on each of them, consecutively:

Ad (1): Since its very beginnings, the British National Health Service (NHS) and its policies have from abroad been looked at as a highly contested medical, social, and ethical experiment. Due to its rather limited budget, NHS has always been known to be in need of denying care to patients on grounds of ressource scarcity. The more, for instance, German experts have become aware of the inevitability to also ration German medical care, the more they have thus been taking an interest in NHS's cutting care policies. One obstacle in taking a serious interest has been the fact that the British health care budget has until now been substantially underfed, thus resulting in a below-European standard of care (e. g. in terms of child mortality or cancer survival – cf. Bericht). But of course this is a contingent fact to be separated from the issue of rationing criteria. In this regard, two points have mainly been critizised: the "ageism" and the coveredness of British rationing. "No dialysis beyond 60" and physicians' pretending medical ineffectiveness when in fact they denied care according to whatever rationing criteria (cf. Aaron and Schwartz) have widely been taken as ethically unjustified, to put it mildly.

As we all know, there are now both dialysis and kidney transplants available in Britain well beyond age 60. Moreover, the British government has recently decided to drastically increase its health care budget, thereby decreasing the extent to which care has to be denied to patients. In this regard, there won't be so much of a difference any more to other European countries. Rather, they face comparable pressures to come to grips with ressource scarcity. Given that Britain has a much longer history of coping and quarreling with the locus and the criteria of rationing decisions, what's the lesson here?

From what we have been told, rationing decisions have predominantly been made by central health authorities under the cover of euphemism and medicalism ("cutting ineffective care"). However, most recent policies tend towards more explicit and decentralized decision making. I was surprised to learn about a whole spectrum of innovative instruments (such as "deliberative opinion polls, mediation groups, referenda and electronic town meetings", "citizens' juries" or "focus groups" p 44) to be in use. In addition, the two recently set-up national institutions (NICE and CHI, see pp 41 ff) have been charged with the production and surveillance of explicit criteria for rationing care. Since those trends are a reaction to critical British debates, we can now turn to level (2) of my above pattern.

Ad (2): Much in line with the aforementioned abroad objections, British critics too have objected to their system's medical paternalism, to the lack of explicit criteria, and to a deficit of democracy in the decision procedures. Hence, there is no need to "enlighten" health policy makers across the Channel with respect to their moral responsibilities. Which criteria have so far been endorsed – for example in framing recommendations by NICE and CH? Guidelines in accord with evidence-based medicine (EBM) – "a technical fix" solution, as Professor Hunter has rightly diagnosed. Without some explicit or implicit criteria for balancing numbers, weighing competing needs, and spelling out, which trade-offs are to be considered fair, EBM won't give sufficient action guidance.

But there are other suggestions, notably supported by the Rationing Agenda Group, namely putting first priority on "unpredictability" and "fundamental importance of the care" considered (pp 42 f). As has been illustrated to us with the example of IVF, the last criterium is prone to very controversial interpretation. The turn to public participation fares no better: lobbyism, bias to seemingly hard numbers, and irrational decision making are among the pitfalls we have learned about. What's the lesson, this time? Professor Hunter's answers are as clear as provocative – and have us turn to level (3) above.

Ad (3): Based on both national experience and international debate, Hunter questions the workability, societal benefit, and thus rationality of explicit rationing as well as the availability of publically acceptable *substantial* criteria of distributive justice in health care. Sharply aware of arguing against "the spirit of the times" he pleas for "muddling through elegantly". This approach, we have learned, would be a combination of central "clinical judgment" and "local discretion" in individual treatment decisions. The latter is to be performed by a participating public; and the whole decision making system is to be framed by very general ethical principles allegedly already backing NHS and by what Hunter calls "procedural rights" (that is rights of patients to have their case reviewed, to be treated without bias, to be given reasons and others). Is this pessimistic but allegeldly "pragmatically sensible" solution acceptable? Is it justified?

Posing Questions

I do not have an answer yet, but rather several open questions. First of all, to many of us who belong to or sympathize with the party Hunter calls the "rational rationer" opponents, his experience- and theory-inspired scepticism may come as a shocking surprise. Used to think, that implicitness and "muddling" in rationing are deplorable deficits of ethical reflexion, we have just been given a sophisticatedly *reflected* plea for purposive implicitness. It seems to shift the burden of prove to the rational rationers' side. It's now their turn to prove the availability of workable explicit strategies. Here come, however, my open questions:

(i) Is it convincing, on a practical level of social interaction, that patients – actual and potential ones – swallow moral judgements disguised as clinical ones?

(ii) So far, both Professor Hunter's and my deliberations have been concerned with the crucial question, how priorities should be set *within* budget constraint. However, part of the non-British debate turns (a) upon alternatives and limits to a commonly paid budget, and thus (b) upon the *content* of a basic care package (commonly paid and universally accessible) which would in turn determine the budget size. Mimicking current US-strategies, there has recently come up much German sympathy for neolibertarian arguments in favour of individual choice among differently thick managed-care packages on the market place.

Doesn't any radical criticism – along those lines – come up in the British public towards the socially-funding *premise* of NHS? Especially when people realize the criterial muddle? In this context, it has, however, been interesting to read about the British Medical Association's protest against the "Private Finance Initiative" (see Bericht).

(iii) What will happen to the "muddling" physicians, to their self-understanding, to their image as patient advocates? Will the trust patients put into their doctors erode – as is often being stipulated in the United States in the context of managed care organizations?

(iv) Given the international failure to come up with some substantial and universally acceptable theory of health care justice, the idea of *procedural* justice is increasingly gaining support (cf. Daniels). However, it makes a big difference whether to *combine* principles of substantial justice with such procedural ones, or to *abandon* the idea of substantive justice altogether – as professor Hunter seems ready to do. Are the limits of philosophical argument to this idea already reached?

(v) Looking a bit closer at his "procedural rights", they seem to embrace some mechanisms of appeal and review in addition to a principle of formal justice (treating like cases alike). It does not need much imagination, to conceive of severe conflicts in interpreting the last one and in balancing competing principles of justice that are prima facie intuitively convincing (such as the "worst-off first principle", the "fair chances principle", or the "maximizing efficiency principle"). If the muddling-through-elegantly approach leaves results to intuitive moral ranking on a local micro level, what happens in case of conflict? Is there a conception of democratic representativity in the back of this approach? How is it spelt out?

(vi) Moreover, what exactly does it mean that patients have a procedural "right to reasons" (p 48)? What happens if they find those reasons unconvincing? And doesn't this very right contradict implicitness? Or is the underlying expectation that patients will readily be contented hearing that nobody in a relevantly similar condition would receive the treatment that is to be denied to him or her?

Whatever the answers, Professor Hunter's plea for intentional "muddling through elegantly" has suggested a new option that cannot simply be dismissed by a "rational rationing" *credo*, anymore.

References

Aaron HJ, Schwartz WB (1984) The painful prescription: rationing hospital care. The Brookings Institution, Washington

Bericht: Britischer Ärztetag: Gesundheitspolitisches Stimmungstief (1999) Deutsches Ärzteblatt 96: S. B1569–70

Daniels N et al. (1996) Benchmarks of Fairness for Health care Reform. OUP, New York

II Practices of Rationing in Germany

Rationing in Intensive Care Medicine

Michael Imhoff

1
Introduction

All Western countries are struggling to curb the continuing growth of health care expenditures. Dramatic changes are happening to the health care systems all over the world. There are many reasons for this development. While an in-depth discussion of these problems is beyond the scope of this presentation, it is worth mentioning that areas of advanced, so-called "high-tech", medicine are obvious targets for criticism in this debate.

With their steady growth health care expenditures have become a major economic factor in modern industrialized societies. They make up between 6 and 14 per cent of the gross domestic product (GDP) of most OECD countries (OECD 1999). As explained later we know that intensive care medicine is probably the single most resource consuming specialty in hospital care. Still, in the medical literature there is little explicit information about methods and practices of rationing in intensive care medicine. Looking at both the per capita healthcare expenditure and the number of publications on rationing in intensive care in seven OECD countries it is striking that the countries with the highest (US) and the lowest (UK) expenditures account for about 90 per cent of all publications. Especially in Germany, which is the country with the third highest absolute health care spending, after the US and Japan (OECD 1999), only very few publications on this issue can be found. Therefore, much of this article will remain conceptual with reference to Germany. On the other hand, many insights and concepts from the US and the UK may be useful for the rationing debate in Germany.

In the following this chapter will focus on four core issues of rationing in intensive care medicine:
- The cost of intensive care medicine.
- The current practices of rationing in intensive care medicine as they are perceived by health care professionals.
- The medical decision making process at the point of care in relation to the problems of rationing.
- Improvements in cost effectiveness in intensive care medicine.
  In conclusion a few perspectives for the future will be given.

2
The Cost of Intensive Care Medicine

Without doubt, intensive care medicine belongs to these exposed areas of modern medicine. In different countries between 1.5 and 10 per cent of all hospital beds are intensive care beds. Intensive care in the US accounts for more than 20 per cent of all hospital reimbursements (Kirton et al. 1996). The daily cost of intensive care management in the United Kingdom is 2–5 times greater than that of general ward management (Ridley, Biggam and Stone 1993). Among other factors, due to shortening the lengths of hospital stays, demographic changes, and advances in medical technology and science, it can be anticipated that the proportion of hospital beds and costs for intensive care will significantly increase in the near future. This makes intensive care the obvious target of cost cutting and rationing discussions.

Looking more closely at the cost of intensive care medicine one has to focus on certain disease entities in the cost analysis:

– Cost of death
– Cost of Multiple Organ Failure (MOF)
– Cost of Sepsis

Looking at the cost of our own surgical ICU, a 16-bed unit in a tertiary referral center, over a three year period we compared the total cost (labor and medications) for critically ill patients with and without septic shock. All 2,488 patients were patients after elective or emergency visceral surgery. 328 patients fulfilled the census conference sepsis criteria and showed the cardio-vascular signs of septic shock. The average treatment cost on the ICU was 14,489 Euro for patients with septic shock compared to 2,505 Euro without. For patients with a failure of three or more organs the average treatment cost was even higher with 17,492 Euro.

These numbers compare well with figures from the United Kingdom (Edbrooke et al. 1999), where patients with sepsis were up to ten times more expensive over their entire length of stay on the ICU. This investigation shows that the decisive factor is not the daily cost but the cumulative cost through the excessive length of stay of these septic patients.

Even more interesting is the cumulative resource consumption for these patients. Although patients in septic shock represent only 13.2 per cent of the patients in our surgical ICU, they consume 46.8 per cent of all ICU resources. The 195 patients in MOF (7.8 per cent) still account for 33.6 per cent of all cost in this unit.

The mortality from septic shock and MOF is still very high, between 20 per cent and over 90 per cent. The majority of patients who die on surgical ICUs die from septic shock, MOF, and surgical and non-surgical complications. It has been known for decades that non-survivors consume the largest portion of expenditures in many ICUs. In our example the approximately 10 per cent of patients that die on the ICU do consume about 50 per cent of all resources. In other words, the expenses for non-survivors double the cost of each patient who survives.

These numbers support the notion that patients with serious complications and those who die account for a disproportionate use of resources in the ICU. This can be seen as a liability, but also as a chance to dramatically improve cost effectiveness for the entire ICU by addressing only a relatively small number of patients. Strategies that help to prevent organ complications and organ failure, or to improve the therapy of these disease entities should also have a strong influence on cost. It is also important to note that non-survivors consume a major amount of ICU resources. Resources that may, in theory, more efficiently be used in patients with better prognosis.

3
The Continuum of Care

However, intensive care cannot be seen without the continuum of care. The continuum of care spans the entire process of therapy and care for a patient with one or multiple illnesses (figure 1). It encompasses the different treatment and care units, such as ER, OR, and general ward. Different modalities of diagnostics (lab, imaging, etc.) and treatment are available. Intensive care is only one piece in the process of care, although sometimes a very important piece. Therefore, it cannot be judged independently, but rather the entire process needs to be analyzed. Many decisions relevant to the outcome, acuity, and cost of the critically ill are made before the patient reaches the ICU. Moreover, pre-ICU decisions and management of patients, e.g. in high-risk surgery, determine utility or futility, success or failure, and ultimately cost-effectiveness of intensive care. Therefore, any debate about cost in intensive care needs to assess the entire continuum of care, even the entire health care system.

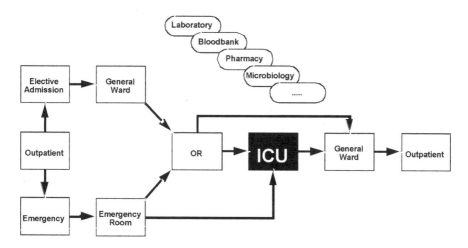

Fig. 1. Schema of the Continuum of Care

4
Practices of Rationing

Even in the richest societies rationing in health care is inevitable and a matter of fact. This has been the case throughout the entire history of medicine. It affects all areas of medicine, including intensive care. Rationing can be achieved in different ways. Various approaches have been implemented in health care:

- Allocating resources to some patients, while denying resources to the treatment of other patients can be seen in many societies, e.g., "rich" vs. "poor". It often results in an allocation of resources according to insurance status. It is not based on medical reasoning and has many ethical, social and political problems.
- Allocating resources to patients following diagnostic, demographic or other medical criteria in order to obtain the greatest benefit for the invested resources is also an old principle of rationing in medicine. This is a standard principle for organ allocation in transplant surgery all over the world. While this principle provides for social equity, at least to some degree, it is dependent on reliable and evidence-based guidelines for the resource allocation. The question is, who will be the final decision maker.
- Global cuts in hospital and health care budgets without redistribution of resources is a principle currently employed in many countries. While this may provide for social equity, it is probably the most inadequate of all rationing principles. In addition to compromising quality of health care it may also slow down medical progress and research. Even investments necessary for quality and efficiency improvements may be impossible under the constraints of tight budgets.

All the above mentioned rationing concepts have multiple drawbacks. They do not provide any form of "intelligent" rationing in the sense of providing for better and more efficient use of scarce health care resources. In clinical practice the rationing may even show a completely different face, many times not overtly but implicit. A few examples from the healthcare professional's "real-world" perspective may highlight this problems the most common practice of implicit rationing are staff reductions and staff limitations for a giving job:

- In the state of Northrhine-Westphalia, Germany, state regulations allow only for a staffing ratio that is significantly below the recommendation of the European Society for Intensive Care Medicine (Ferdinande 1997). For instance, the recommended ratio of nursing staff for a level III ICU to operated beds is 4–6 nursing FTEs to one bed. In reality it is 2.3 to 1, which means that one nurse has to care for about 3 patients simultaneously during a shift (nursing ratio 3:1). The same is true for physicians (40 per cent of the recommendation) or physio-therapists (25 per cent of the recommendations). Recent US studies show that staff reductions may even increase the cost per patient by provoking preventable complications. In one US study with 2,606 patients after abdominal aortic surgery ICUs with a nursing ratio worse than 2:1 had a 50 per cent longer stay per patient, a 4.4 times higher rate of pulmonary insufficiency, a 2.6 times higher rate of reintubation, and a 50 per cent higher rate of cardiac complications when compared to units with a nursing ratio of better than 2:1 (Pronovost, Dang et al. 1999, Pronovost, Jenckes et al. 1999).

– Every winter there is an extreme shortage of ICUs beds in Canada. The reason for this phenomenon is the yearly (and predictable) recurrence of an influenza epidemic. Despite the evident knowledge about this seasonal phenomenon as of today nothing has been done to solve the problem of patient's being denied access to ICUs in Canadian winters (Lomas [in press]).

– Withdrawal or withholding of therapy in intensive care today is the rule rather than the exception in clinical practice. In a recent survey only 23 per cent of the patients dying in ICUs in the US died under full ICU care (Prendergast et al. 1998).

Most of the problems of rationing in clinical practice are related to decision making in health care. Therefore, it appears to be sensible to take a closer look at decision making in intensive care medicine and how decision making practices may actually affect rationing.

5
Decision-Making in Intensive Care Medicine

5.1
Information Overload

An abundance of information is generated during the process of critical care. Much of this information can now be captured and stored using clinical information systems (CIS) which provide for complete medical documentation at the bedside. The clinical usefulness and efficiency of clinical information systems has been proven repeatedly (Imhoff 1995, Imhoff 1996, Imhoff et al. 1994). While databases with more than 2,000 individual patient-related variables are now available for further analysis (Imhoff 1998), the multitude of variables presented at the bedside even without a CIS precludes medical judgement by humans. A physician may be confronted with more than 200 variables in the critically ill during typical morning rounds (Morris and Gardner 1992). However, even an experienced physician is often not able to develop a systematic response to any problem involving more than seven variables (Miller 1956). Moreover, humans are limited in their ability to estimate the degree of relatedness between only two variables (Jennings et al. 1982). This problem is most pronounced in the evaluation of the measurable effect of a therapeutic intervention. Personal bias, experience, and a certain expectation toward the respective intervention may distort an objective judgement (Guyatt et al. 1986).

On the level of the hospital enterprise, information overload is an issue, too. In addition to administrative aspects of such a complex enterprise, new and much more complicated reimbursement and accounting policies lead to an unmatched complexity of data and information (Haux 1997).

The volume of scientific literature is growing exponentially. As of 1993 the number of systematic reviews in medicine increased 500 fold over a ten year period

(Chalmers and Laus 1993). It is impossible for the individual health care professional to keep track of all relevant medical knowledge even in very narrow subspecialities.

5.2
Human (Medical) Errors

Moreover, we know that human errors are unavoidable. They occur infrequently (< 1 per cent), but may compromise patient safety. In the light of the evident information overload they must be regarded as the expression of a systematic fault in the health care delivery system, rather than as an individual shortcoming (Abramson et al. 1980, Leape 1994, Morris 1999, Wu et al. 1991).

Recent studies have reported that the incidence of medication errors for hospital inpatients range from 4 to 10 per cent (Lesar 1997). In a recent study is has been estimated that adverse drug events (ADE), of which about half appear to be preventable, account for 4.8 per cent of per capita care expenditures in those US states where the study was conducted (Thomas et al. 1999). For US inpatient encounters a rate of 6.5 ADEs per 100 non-obstetric admissions has been reported of which 12 per cent were life-threatening and 1 per cent fatal (Bates et al. 1995).

Although it can be expected that in intensive care units, especially in closed units, continuous intensivist presence, special education, and highly trained nurses may limit the occurrence and effects of adverse drug events, this issue of medication errors may have a significant impact on outcome and cost effectiveness in the treatment of patients with sepsis and MOF. This assumption is supported by a study into critical care outcome that showed that iatrogenic adverse events, most often ADEs, were among the three variables most strongly associated with unfavourable ICU outcome (Ferraris/Propp 1992).

These arguments motivate the use of decision support systems. Clinical decision support aims at providing health care professionals with therapy guidelines directly at the point of care. This should enhance the quality of clinical care, since the guidelines sort out high value practices from those that have little or no value. The goal of decision support is to supply the best recommendation under all circumstances (Morris 1998).

5.3
The Evidence of best Medical Practice

But even if all therapeutic interventions are performed following guidelines and protocols, the question is not easy to answer whether these guidelines actually represent the best possible medical practice. This problem is by far not specific for the treatment of the critically ill. The majority of all medical interventions, according to some authors up to 85 per cent, are not supported by clinical data that show that these interventions do more good than harm (Morris 1999). Treatments and even guidelines based on uncontrolled clinical experience bear the danger of being widely applied, even if they are useless or harmful (Cook 1994, Guyatt et al. 1993). Recent studies suggest that, depending on country and health care systems, up to 50 per cent of hospital care is not clinically warranted (Axene 1994).

6
Improvements in Cost Effectiveness

6.1
Goals

The ideal solution would be a method that allows the reduction of health care costs and at the same time provides for improved quality of care and better outcomes. Although this sounds like a dream this goal could be achieved with consistency in the implementation of decision-making support and standardization in the process of care. The key is how information is managed and how decisions are made particularly at the bedside and in general throughout the continuum of care.

This goal may be achieved by the following measures:

– Standardization of care leading to a reduction of intra- and inter-individual variance of care.
– Development of standards and guidelines following rational principles.
– Continuous control and validation of standards and guidelines against new scientific evidence and against actual patient data.

6.2
Controlling the Process of Care

The use of guidelines, protocols, and algorithms in clinical practice can improve patient outcome (Grimm et al. 1975, Grimshaw and Russell 1993, Morris 1999, Wirtschafter et al. 1981). Numerous studies and reviews have shown this (Grimshaw and Russell 1993). A large meta-analysis found in the majority of studies significant improvements in patient outcome through the implementation of computer-based decision support (Johnston et al. 1994). It should be noted that none of the investigated systems featured a complete electronic patient record.

Even without the use of sophisticated computer systems, protocols can significantly improvement patient care (Grimm 1975).

Point-of-care information systems allow the broadest control over the process of care. Outstanding examples for the control and management of the process control level are computerized protocols (overview in: Morris 1999), clinical pathways, and guidelines.

Order entry and decision support systems offer a unique opportunity to dramatically improve the quality of care while at the same time reducing overall costs (Classen et al. 1992, Pestotnik et al. 1996). In the terminology of total quality management (TQM), an explicit method, e.g., a computerized protocol, is part of the stabilization of the process necessary to improve quality (Shewart 1931, Walton 1986).

6.3
Clinical Pathways

A clinical pathway can be defined as an outline of services and therapies for a typical patient with a specific diagnosis. Clinical pathways provide the formal structure for the standardization of care throughout the entire process of care for common diagnoses and treatments.

Numerous studies on the impact of clinical pathways in the process of care can be found. Only in the last couple of years have several dozen clinical studies been done to assess improvements of cost effectiveness and outcome by clinical pathways. Most of these studies span the entire continuum of care, at least during one hospital stay (selection of studies in table 1, p 72). Some studies focus more specifically on intensive care (selection of studies in table 2, p 73).

All studies have a serious short coming in that the protocol groups are compared to historic control cohorts. On the other hand, nearly all studies show marked reductions in cost and length of stay. Deterioration of outcome is never reported. In some studies even outcome measures, such as rate of complications or hospital survival, improve. Except for one (Chang et al. 1999) all studies were done in the US. Therefore, one should be cautious to extrapolate the cost benefits directly to European health care, because of the different cost structures. On the other hand it is quite obvious that medical improvements, such as reduction in the length of stay or improvements in complication rate and outcome can also be achieved in other health care systems.

Also the studies that focus on intensive care need to be seen in the perspective of the entire continuum of care. This is most obvious in the study by Back et al. (Back et al. 1997) where the largest cost benefit stems from preventing ICU admission in the course of elective surgery. It shows the importance of pre-ICU decisions and treatment for the actual success and cost of intensive care. Simple things that may be part of a pathway like the testing and replenishing of blood potassium levels prior to cardiac surgery (Wahr et al. 1999) may have a dramatic effect on post-operative intensive care. On the other hand, the early admission of patients to the ICU for hemodynamic optimization may significantly improve outcome and reduce cost (Wilson et al. 1999). Therefore, it is necessary to develop clinical pathways for the entire continuum of care, as this will have the strongest impact on the overall cost effectiveness and outcome. This approach may also help to limit cases of futile intensive care medicine and make scant ICU beds available for those who benefit most. But even on the micro level clinical pathways provide a tool to improve the quality and cost efficiency of intensive care (Marx et al. 1999).

6.4
Computerized Protocols

There are different levels of clinical decision support. Many systems that implement medical guidelines or clinical pathways are time oriented rather than patient data driven. This contrasts to computerized protocols where actual patient data generates executable instructions (recommendations) on the bases of validated rules (Classen et al. 1992, Classen et al. 1997, East 1994, Morris 1999, Pestotnik et al. 1996).

The most detailed and explicit algorithms in clinical decision making use rule-based computer systems (Johnston et al. 1994, Morris 1999). Electronic reminders can significantly improve physicians' compliance with guidelines, reduce the rate of human errors and make physicians more responsive to specific clinical events (McDonald 1976, McDonald et al. 1980).

Using data from the most comprehensive singular clinical data repository at the LDS Hospital, Salt Lake City, Utah, USA, the group of Morris (Thomsen et al. 1993) developed a rule-based DSS for the mechanical ventilation of the critically ill, which generates, on the basis of actual patient data, explicit, executable and reproducible instructions or recommendations for the next therapeutic step. It was possible to control more than 95 per cent of the ventilation times with these protocols, while intermediate and final clinical outcomes showed a beneficial effect (Morris 1999).

When a decision support system checked all doctor's orders for drug interactions, of 15,000 daily orders approximately 400 were changed in a large US institution, mostly for potential adverse drug events (Teich et al. 1999). It has even been estimated that manual paper-based screening for in-hospital adverse drug effects detects only about 5 per cent of all events that can be detected with computerized systems (Classen et al. 1997).

On the basis of broad clinical experience it can be said that clinical care with bedside computerized protocols is feasible. Moreover, it complies with the ethical imperatives of modern health care (Morris 1998, Sharpe and Faden 1998).

6.5
Evidence-Based Medicine

Evidence-based methods help to generate rule-bases by integrating high-quality clinical research evidence with pathophysiological reasoning, care-giver experience, and patient preferences (Cook 1998). While this level of scientific and societal information does not provide direct control of the process of care, it fulfills an important task: With the help of EBM it allows developing guidelines and pathways with strong scientific foundations. It can select concepts that have been proven to do more good than harm. In that respect, EBM can significantly contribute to improve cost-effectiveness of the process of care.

The knowledge in the societal and epidemiological domains determines the framework of medicine. EBM provides us with methods and concepts to extract and validate the scientific information relevant for the process of care from the vastness of scientific literature.

6.6
The Implementation of Clinical Pathways and Protocols
in Clinical Practice

After the development of a clinical pathway or a protocol, its implementation into clinical practice is the next essential step. For successful and consistent use of a protocol

– the users must be aware of the protocol,

– the protocol must be available wherever it is needed, i.e., at the point-of-care,
– the protocol must be accessible when it is required,
– the user needs to be reminded when action is required according to the protocol.

These requirements are nearly impossible to fulfill with a paper-based clinical pathway. In particular, automatic reminders and ubiquitous availability cannot be achieved. Therefore, consistent use of a clinical pathway only appears feasible with the help of point-of-care information systems (Bates et al. 1998, Teich et al. 1999). The electronic patient record is the ideal vehicle for clinical pathways, as it also allows the comprehensive data acquisition for validation and quality control of pathways.

7
Implications for the Rationing Debate

Health care expenditures are an important economical factor in every industrialized country. Intensive care medicine is among the most expensive specialties. Therefore, intensive care medicine is an obvious target in the rationing debate.

In intensive care medicine but also in all other areas of health care there is a significant potential to improve quality of care and at the same time to save money by employing clinical decision support and advanced healthcare information technology.

The imperative of rationing is first to exploit all opportunities for rationalization before rationing the respective good. In this respect improvements of cost effectiveness and quality in healthcare are the prerequisites for rational rationing. Currently rationing in healthcare is not obeying this imperative at all. Rationing in healthcare and also in intensive care is implicitly practiced every day in hospitals all over the world. Still, little is done, at least in Europe to improve cost effectiveness and quality of care on a broad scale. There are many, often irrational reasons for this, and their discussion goes beyond the scope of this presentation.

Major improvements in cost effectiveness are feasible. This can lift the pressure on health care expenditures significantly. It will not make rationing unnecessary, but it will enable us to provide better care to more people at the same expense.

Of course, this does not answer all ethical, philosophical, legal, and macro economical questions. But it may help to make rational and politically, socially and ethically acceptable decisions.

8
References

Abramson NS, Wald KS, Grenvik AN, Robinson D, Snyder JV (1980) Adverse occurrences in intensive care units. JAMA 244, pp 1582–1584

Axene D, Doyle R (1994) Analysis of medically unnecessary inpatient service. Research Report. Milliman & Robertson, Seattle

Back MR, Harward TR, Huber TS, Carlton LM, Flynn TC, Seeger JM (1997) Improving the cost-effectiveness of carotid endarterectomy. J Vasc Surg 26, pp 456–462

Bates DW, Cullen DJ, Laird N, Petersen LA, Small SD, Servi D, Laffel G, Sweitzer BJ, Shea BF, Hallisey R (1995) Incidence of adverse drug events and potential adverse drug events. Implications for prevention. ADE Prevention Study Group. JAMA 274, pp 29–34

Bates DW, Pappius EM, Kuperman GJ, Sittig D, Burstin H, Fairchild D, Brennan TA, Teich JM (1998) Measuring and improving quality using information systems. Medinfo 9 Pt 2, pp 814–818

Burns SM, Marshall M, Burns JE, Ryan B, Wilmoth D, Carpenter R, Aloi A, Wood M, Truwit JD (1998) Design, testing, and results of an outcomes-managed approach to patients requiring prolonged mechanical ventilation. Am J Crit Care 7, pp 45–57

Chalmers TC, Laus J (1993) Meta-analytic stimulus for changes in clinical trials. Stat Methods Med Res 2, pp 161–172

Chang PL, Wang TM, Huang ST, Hsieh ML, Tsui KH, Lai RH (1999) Effects of implementation of 18 clinical pathways on costs and quality of care among patients undergoing urological surgery. J Urol 161, pp 1858–1862

Classen DC, Evans RS, Pestotnik SL, Horn SD, Menlove RL, Burke JP (1992) The timing of prophylactic administration of antibiotics and the risk of surgical-wound infection. N Engl J Med 326, pp 281–286

Classen DC, Pestotnik SL, Evans RS, Lloyd JF, Burke JP (1997) Adverse drug events in hospitalized patients. Excess length of stay, extra costs, and attributable mortality. JAMA 277, pp 301–306

Cook D (1994) Small trials in critical care medicine: What can intensivists learn from them? In: Vincent JL (ed) Yearbook of Intensive and Emergency Medicine 1994. Springer, Berlin pp 779–785

Cook D (1998) Evidence-based critical care medicine. A potential tool for change. New Horizons 6, pp 20–25

Dzwierzynski WW, Spitz K, Hartz A, Guse C, Larson DL (1998) Improvement in resource utilization after development of a clinical pathway for patients with pressure ulcers. Plast Reconstr Surg 102, pp 2006–2011

East T (1994) Role of the computer in the delivery of mechanical ventilation. In: Tobin M (ed) Principles and Practice of Mechanical Ventilation. MacGraw-Hill, New York, pp 1005–1038

Edbrooke DL, Hibbert CL, Kingsley JM, Smith S, Bright NM, Quinn JM (1999) The patient-related cost of care for sepsis patients in a United Kingdom adult general intensive care unit. Crit Care Med 27, pp 1760–1767

Ferdinande P (1997) Recommendations on minimal requirements for Intensive Care Departments. Members of the Task Force of the European Society of Intensive Care Medicine. Intensive Care Med 23, pp 226–232

Ferraris VA, Propp ME (1992) Outcome in critical care patients: a multivariate study. Crit Care Med 20, pp 967–976

Gandhi RR, Keller MS, Schwab CW, Stafford PW (1999) Pediatric splenic injury: pathway to play? J Pediatr Surg 34, pp 55–58

Gheiler EL, Lovisolo JA, Tiguert R, Tefilli MV, Grayson T, Oldford G, Powell IJ, Famiglietti G, Banerjee M, Pontes JE, Wood DP Jr. (1999) Results of a clinical care pathway for radical prostatectomy patients in an open hospital – multiphysician system. Eur Urol 35, pp 210–216

Grimm RH Jr., Shimoni K, Harlan WR Jr., Estes EH Jr. (1975) Evaluation of patient-care protocol use by various providers. N Engl J Med 292, pp 507–511

Grimshaw JM, Russell IT (1993) Effect of clinical guidelines on medical practice: a systematic review of rigorous evaluations. Lancet 342, pp 1317–1322

Guyatt G, Drummond M, Feeny D, Tugwell P, Stoddart G, Haynes RB, Bennett K, Labelle R (1986) Guidelines for the clinical and economic evaluation of health care technologies. Soc Sci Med 22, pp 393–408

Guyatt GH, Sackett DL, Cook DJ (1993) Users' guides to the medical literature. II. How to use an article about therapy or prevention. A. Are the results of the study valid? Evidence-Based Medicine Working Group. JAMA 270, pp 2598–2601

Haux R (1997) Aims and tasks of medical informatics. Int J Med Inf 44, pp 9–20

Imhoff M (1995) A clinical information system on the intensive care unit: dream or night mare? In: Rubi JAG (ed) Medicina Intensiva 1995, XXX. Congreso SEMIUC. Murcia. Pictographia, Murcia, pp 17–22

Imhoff M (1996) 3 years clinical use of the Siemens Emtek System 2000: Efforts and Benefits. Clinical Intensive Care 7 (Suppl.), pp 43–44

Imhoff M, Lehner JH, Löhlein D (1994) 2 years clinical experience with a clinical information system on a surgical ICU. In: Mutz NJ, Koller W, Benzer H (eds) 7th European Congress on Intensive Care Medicine. Monduzi Editore, Bologna, pp 163–166

Imhoff M (1998) Clinical Data Acquisition: What and how? Journal für Anästhesie und Intensivmedizin 5, pp 85–86

Jennings D, Amabile T, Ross L (1982) Informal covariation assessments: Data-based versus theory-based judgements. In: Kahnemann D, Slovic P, Tversky A (eds) Judgement under uncertainty: Heuristics and biases. Cambridge University Press, Cambridge, pp 211–230

Johnston ME, Langton KB, Haynes RB, Mathieu A (1994) Effects of computer-based clinical decision support systems on clinician performance and patient outcome. A critical appraisal of research. Ann Intern Med 120, pp 135–142

Kirton OC, Civetta JM, Hudson-Civetta J (1996) Cost effectiveness in the intensive care unit. Surg Clin North Am 7, pp 175–200

Leape L (1994) Error in medicine. JAMA 272, pp 1851–1857

Lesar TS, Briceland L, Stein DS (1997) Factors related to errors in medication prescribing. JAMA 277, pp 312–317

Lomas J (in press) Health Services Research. In: Sibbald W, Bion J (eds) Evaluating Critical Care: Using health services research to improve quality. Update in Intensive Care and Emergency Medicine. Springer, Heidelberg

Marx WH, DeMaintenon NL, Mooney KF, Mascia ML, Medicis J, Franklin PD, Sivak E, Rotello L (1999) Cost reduction and outcome improvement in the intensive care unit. J Trauma 46, pp 625–30

McDonald CJ (1976) Protocol-based computer reminders, the quality of care and the non-perfectability of man. N Engl J Med 295, pp 1351–1355

McDonald CJ, Wilson GA, McCabe GP Jr. (1980) Physician response to computer reminders. JAMA 244, pp 1579–1581

Miller G (1956) The magical number seven, plus of minus two: Some limits to our capacity for processing information. Psychol Rev 63, pp 81–97

Morris A, Gardner R (1992) Computer applications. In: Hall J, Schmidt G, Wood L (eds) Principles of Critical Care. McGraw-Hill, New York, pp 500–514

Morris A (1998) Algorithm-Based Decision-Making. In: Tobin JA (ed) Principles and Practice of Intensive Care Monitoring. McGraw-Hill, New York, pp 1355–1381

Morris AH (1999) Computerized protocols and beside decision support. Crit Care Clin 15, pp 523–545

OECD (1999) OECD Health Data 1999: A Comparative Analysis of 29 Countries

Pestotnik SL, Classen DC, Evans RS, Burke JP (1996) Implementing antibiotic practice guidelines through computer-assisted decision support: clinical and financial outcomes. Ann Intern Med 124, pp 884–890

Price MB, Jones A, Hawkins JA, McGough EC, Lambert L, Dean JM (1999) Critical pathways for postoperative care after simple congenital heart surgery. Am J Manag Care 5, pp 185–192

Prendergast TJ, Claessens MT, Luce JM (1998) A national survey of end-of-life care for critically ill patients. Am J Respir Crit Care Med 158, pp 1163–1167

Pronovost PJ, Dang D, Dorman T, Jenckes MW, Garrett E, Bass EB (1999) ICU nurse to patient ratio greater than 1 to 2 associated with an increased risk of complications in abdominal aortic surgery. Crit Care Med 27 (Suppl.) A27

Pronovost PJ, Jenckes MW, Dorman T, Garrett E, Breslow MJ, Rosenfeld BA, Lipsett PA, Bass E (1999) Organizational characteristics of intensive care units related to outcomes of abdominal aortic surgery. JAMA 281, pp 1310–1317

Ridley S, Biggam M, Stone P (1993) A cost-benefit analysis of intensive therapy. Anaesthesia 48, pp 14–19

Scranton PE Jr. (1999) The cost effectiveness of streamlined care pathways and product standardization in total knee arthroplasty. J Arthroplasty 14, pp 182–186

Sharpe V, Faden A (1998) Medical Harm. Cambridge University Press, Cambridge, UK

Shewart W (1931) Economic control of quality of manufactured product. D. Van Nostrand New York

Spain DA, McIlvoy LH, Fix SE, Carrillo EH, Boaz PW, Harpring JE, Raque GH, Miller FB (1998) Effect of a clinical pathway for severe traumatic brain injury on resource utilization. J Trauma 45, pp 101–104

Teich JM, Glaser JP, Beckley RF, Aranow M, Bates DW, Kuperman GJ, Ward ME, Spurr CD (1999) The Brigham integrated computing system (BICS) advanced clinical systems in an academic hospital environment. Int J Med Inf 54, pp 197–208

Thomas EJ, Studdert DM, Newhouse JP, Zbar BI, Howard KM, Williams EJ, Brennan TA (1999) Cost of medical injuries in Utah and Colorado. Inquiry 36, pp 255–264

Thomsen GE, Pope D, East TD, Morris AH, Kinder AT, Carlson DA, Smith GL, Wallace CJ, Orme JF Jr., Clemmer TP (1993) Clinical performance of a rule-based decision support system for mechanical ventilation of ARDS patients. Proc Annu Symp Comput Appl Med Care 1993, pp 339–343

Uzark K, Frederick C, Lamberti JJ, Worthen HM, Ogino MT, Mainwaring RD, Moore JW (1998) Changing practice patterns for children with heart disease: a clinical pathway approach. Am J Crit Care 7, pp 101–105

Velasco FT, Ko W, Rosengart T, Altorki N, Lang S, Gold JP, Krieger KH, Isom OW (1996) Cost containment in cardiac surgery: results with a critical pathway for coronary bypass surgery at the New York hospital-Cornell Medical Center. Best Pract Benchmarking Healthc 1, pp 21–28

Wahr JA, Parks R, Boisvert D, Comunale M, Fabian J, Ramsay J, Mangano DT (1999) Preoperative serum potassium levels and perioperative outcomes in cardiac surgery patients. JAMA 281, pp 2203–2210

Walton M (1986) The Deming management method. Putnam, New York

Warner BW, Kulick RM, Stoops MM, Mehta S, Stephan M, Kotagal UR (1998) An evidenced-based clinical pathway for acute appendicitis decreases hospital duration and cost. J Pediatr Surg 33, pp 1371–1375

Wilson J, Woods I, Fawcett J, Whall R, Dibb W, Morris C, McManus E (1999) Reducing the risk of major elective surgery: randomised controlled trial of preoperative optimisation of oxygen delivery. BMJ 318, pp 1099–1103

Wirtschafter DD, Scalise M, Henke C, Gams RA (1981) Do information systems improve the quality of clinical research? Results of a randomized trial in a cooperative multi-institutional cancer group. Comput Biomed Res 14, pp 78–90

Wu AW, Folkman S, McPhee SJ, Lo B (1991) Do house officers learn from their mistakes? JAMA 265, pp 2089–2094

Zehr KJ, Dawson PB, Yang SC, Heitmiller RF (1998) Standardized clinical care pathways for major thoracic cases reduce hospital costs. Ann Thorac Surg 66, pp 914–919

9
Tables

Table 1. Clinical Pathway studies across the continuum of care

Publication	Clinical Setting	N	Efficiency	Outcome
Chang et al., 1999 [8]	Urological surgery	protocol: 1,382 control (historic): 1,279	Hospital LOS[1]: −11 per cent (p < 0.05)	Reduction of postoperative complications
Dzwierzynski et al., 1998 [13]	Pressure ulcer therapy	protocol: 43 control (historic): 52	Total cost: −23 per cent (p < 0.05)	no change
Gheiler et al., 1999 [19]	Radical prostatectomy	total: 1,129	Hospital LOS: −34 per cent (p < 0.05)	no change
Scranton, 1998 [49]	Total knee arthroplasty	protocol: 77 control (historic): 52	Hospital LOS: −37 per cent (p < 0.05) Hospital charges: − US$ 1,063	no change
Warner et al., 1998 [60]	Pediatric appendicitis	protocol: 120 control (historic): 122	Hospital LOS: −39 per cent (p < 0.05) Hospital costs: −30 per cent (p < 0.05)	no change
Zehr et al., 1998 [64]	Esophagectomy	protocol: 96 control (historic): 56	Hospital LOS: −30 per cent (p < 0.05) Hospital charges: −34 per cent (p < 0.05)	slightly reduced mortality (n.s.)
Zehr et al., 1998 [64]	Lung resection	protocol: 241 control (historic): 185	Hospital LOS: −20 per cent (p < 0.05) Hospital charges: −21 per cent (p < 0.05)	no change

---

[1] LOS = length of stay

Table 2. Clinical Pathway studies explicitly involving intensive care

Publication	Clinical Setting	N	Efficiency	Outcome
Back et al., 1997 [3]	ICU admissions for carotid endarterectomy	protocol: 63 control (historic): 45	ICU admissions: −70 per cent (p < 0.05) Total costs: −41 per cent (p < 0.05)	no change
Burns et al., 1998 [6]	Prolonged mechanical ventilation	protocol: 90 control (historic): 124	Vent days: −1.3 days (n.s.) Hospital LOS: −2.1 days (n.s.) Total costs: −US$ 3,341 per case	no change
Gandhi et al., 1999 [18]	Pediatric blunt splenic injury	protocol: 21 control (historic): 28	ICU LOS: −28 per cent (n.s.) hospital LOS: −21 per cent (p < 0.05)	no change
Price et al., 1999 [44]	Pediatric cardiac surgery	protocol: 46 control (historic): 58	ICU LOS: −50 per cent (p < 0.05) hospital LOS: −40 per cent (p < 0.05) cost: −49 per cent (p < 0.05)	no change
Spain et al., 1998 [52]	Severe head injuries	protocol: 84 control (historic): 49	Vent. days: −21 per cent (p < 0.05) ICU LOS: −21 per cent (p < 0.05) Hospital LOS: −24 per cent (p < 0.05, only calculated for survivors)	no change in functional outcome or complications, higher mortality throug end-of-life decisions by family members

Publication	Clinical Setting	N	Efficiency	Outcome
Uzark et al., 1998 [56]	Pediatric cardiac surgery	protocol: 173 control: 69	Vent days: −40 per cent (p < 0.05) Lab tests: −25 per cent Total costs: −20 per cent	no change
Velasco et al., 1996 [57]	Adult cardiac surgery	protocol: 114 control (historic): 382	ICU LOS: −46 per cent (p < 0.05) Hospital LOS: −31 per cent (p < 0.05) Total costs: −US $ 1,181 (p < 0.05)	no change

Global Budgets and Rationing

Rationing is inevitable:
Modern Medicine as a Victim of its own Success

Walter Krämer

What makes rationing in the context of global budgets different from rationing in other contexts? What is so peculiar about the interplay between the two? The answer is: not very much.

Still, there are some aspects which deserve attention: For instance, global budgets are a forceful reminder to the health industry and to the public at large that medical resources are finite. To an economist, and in fact to almost everybody else except German health professionals, this might seem a truth too obvious to be worth discussing. May I remind the reader that until quite recently, it was considered unethical by most German physicians to even think of not completely exhausting the range of the medically feasible. These days are gone, and global budgets have helped a lot in driving home the fact that resources will never be sufficient to support an expansion of the supply of medical care up to the point where marginal utility is zero.

However, there is a second aspect to the rationing-and-global-budgets-issue which I think is more important. This is that global budgets brake up the rationing process into two major stages, and that different principles apply at each of these stages.

Stage one (which has also been called the macro stage) concerns the decision: How many resources is society as a whole willing and able to spend on medical care? At this stage, no individual patients are involved. Of course, limiting resources at this stage will eventually lead to premature deaths and lost years of life, but the individuals who are involved are not known at the time the decision is taken. Decisions at this stage involve the killing of statistical lives, so to speak.

This is a point of utmost importance! Rationing at the global budget level does not kill individual people; it only affects *survival probabilities*, and this is an extremely important difference! In particular, and other than individual lives, survival probabilities can easily be priced and traded on the market.

For instance, to mention a famous brand of cars that has been referred to several times today, do you know that about 1,000 people die on the streets in Germany each year because they do *not* drive a Mercedes-Benz? Not driving a Mercedes-Benz implies a considerable reduction in survival probabilities. Still, many people think that buying this extra survival probability is not worth the money. And so far, I have not heart of any plans to make a Mercedes-Benz available to every German through the health car system.

By the same token, devoting 500 billion rather than 600 billion Deutschmarks per year to medical care involves a certain reduction in survival probabilities for most members of the population, but this reduction is as ethically defensible as not buying a Mercedes Benz.

There is another lesson to be learnt from this: that the principle of rationing by killing statistical rather than individual lives should be followed as far down the road as possible. Given that it is ethically more acceptable to ration medical care by reducing survival probabilities rather than to ration it by denying care to identifiable individuals, this principle appears to me to be the ideal way out of the moral dilemma involved in rationing modern medicine.

Some Examples

I stumbled across an article entitled "Unrentables Gegengift" in the German newspaper *DIE ZEIT* when I was preparing my remarks. The article is about some very costly anti-snake-vaccine which is no longer being produced. The article goes on to state that in some regions of Africa, thousands of people die each year from snake bites because this vaccine is no longer available. Apart from the fact that this affair is taking place in Africa and not in Central Europe: Does society have the moral duty to continue producing this type of medication? I think not! However, if this vaccine is available at all, then it should be administered to everybody who needs it. The principle question is: Should it or should it not be available in the first place?

Many decisions in health care planning are of this type: whether or not to implement an emergency helicopter system in some sparsely populated area (there was a major public outrage when sick funds in Bavaria declined to pay for such a system in the area of Regensburg), whether or not to establish facilities for organ transplantation, whether or not to continue research into artificial hearts or microsurgery or anti-AIDS-drugs and so forth. The common denominator of all these decision problems is that it is only survival probabilities and not identifiable individuals which are at stake. And as long as rationing is taking place in this space of survival probabilities, I have little trouble with it.

Global Budgets and Rationing

Rationing in Medicine:
Some Issues in the Light of Economic Theory

Peter Zweifel

This contribution is about three issues surrounding rationing in medicine that readily come to the mind of a person that has an economic background. For economic theory has much to say about the advantages (and disadvantages) of different rationing mechanisms, among them markets and market prices in particular. It considers rationing imposed by governments as an inferior alternative, one that a nation may resort to in wartime. In times of war, many goods become very scarce in supply, so their market price would skyrocket, putting them out of reach of many consumers and lavishing windfall gains on suppliers. To prevent this from happening, governments use rationing as a quick fix, seeking to stave off social unrest at a time when the nation is struggling for survival. This characterization of rationing gives rise to provocative thoughts such as: Are today's industrial countries waging a war in their health care sectors? Against whom? Are physicians and hospitals about to reap huge windfall gains due to skyrocketing fees for their services?

Even without exploring the parallels with wartime rationing any further, three specific issues that have implications for the ethics of rationing in medicine seem worthwhile to be considered, viz (1) a comparison of the criteria of evaluation applied by consumers and politicians for the ranking and allocation of scarce health care services; (2) the fact that self-rationing occurs in everyday life and that insurance plans may be used to induce self-rationing in health care; and (3) the problem of bad decisions in the choice of such insurance plans.

1
Comparison of Criteria of Evaluation Applied by Consumers and Politicians

In everyday life, individuals seek to obtain "value for money". In economic terms, they compare the benefits with the costs (which actually need not only be financial but may include time and effort spent in obtaining the good or service as well) when deciding whether or not to demand (more of) a particular good or service. This means that consumers may be prepared to spend a great deal of money if they judge the benefits important enough. More to the point, in everyday life people do not minimize cost or expenditure, or else they would all be driving the cheapest cars available (or rely on public transportation altogether); luxury cars would be entirely absent from the streets.

Now when justifying rationing in health care, politicians invariably claim that health care takes too much of people's income, or more technically, the country's Gross National Product (GNP). Apparently, they seek ways to reduce health care expenditure – but how do they know that this is in the interest of consumers? After all, many consumers might achieve their highest ratio of benefit to cost at a still higher (rather than lower) level of health care expenditure!

Indeed, it is easy to see why politicians would want to emphasize the expenditure rather than the benefit side of the ratio. Up until rather recently, they were able to win elections promising "Health for All By the Year X" (the World Health Organization used to put X = 2000 but had to face the fact that this target is unrealistic). Now given that a politician has indeed won an election, he or she has every interest in fulfilling this promise at the lowest possible cost to her or him. Clearly, this differs from the cost borne by the consumers in the guise of taxes, insurance contributions, and out-of-pocket payments in the event of illness. To a politician, the true cost of health care is that part of the public budget which is tied to health and therefore is not available for obtaining votes from pivotal constituencies (by paying out subsidies to farmers, providing building contracts to the construction industry and defense contracts to the machine and electronics industries, e.g.).

This difference of criteria used for evaluation (i.e. ranking goods and services as more or less important in the context of rationing) raises the question: What is ethically recommendable about letting politicians impose their emphasis on just the expenditure part of the benefit-cost ratio in health?

2
Self-Rationing in Everyday Life and the Use of Insurance Plans to Induce Self-Rationing in Health Care

Outside the health care sector, individuals ration themselves every day. Applying the benefit-cost-ratio criterion expounded in the previous paragraph, consumers continually settle for less than would be available in principle. For example, they do drive cars that specialized magazines would not recommend, judging them to be of inferior quality. However, their user cost in terms of operation, depreciation, and maintenance may be so low that the benefit-cost ratio looks excellent to at least some consumers.

By way of contrast, only the very best seems to be good enough when it comes to health care. From the economic point of view, this is not astonishing at all but can be interpreted as the natural consequence of (almost) complete insurance coverage. With complete insurance coverage, the financial cost of treatment to a patient is simply zero regardless of whether he or she opts for the latest (and usually most expensive) medical technology or not. As soon as the new technology offers better treatment alternatives and/or causes less pain or inconvenience, the choice is clear: it is preferred regardless of actual cost. The very small copayments required in most of today's health care systems do not modify this conclusion appreciably. In particular, there is accumulating evidence to the effect that the latest and most expensive medical technology comes to use precisely during the last few months of human life, at a time where most patients presumably can guess that their chance of survival is low.

Patients would ration themselves if they derived an advantage from it. In everyday life, this advantage amounts to the money saved by e. g. driving a car of less than superb quality. In the context of health care, the advantage of making do without the latest medical technology could be lower contributions to health insurance. Indeed, health insurers estimate that limiting benefits to cover technology that is at least five years old may reduce medical expenditure by 20 per cent or more. Insureds could therefore ration themselves by signing up for a plan that gave them a premium reduction of (say) 30 per cent if they agreed to having it exclude the latest technology beyond age 50, of 20 per cent beyond age 60, and 10 per cent beyond age 70.

This possibility gives rise to another question, viz: What is ethically objectionable about offering individuals health insurance plans that exclude the latest medical technology in return for a reduced contribution?

3
The Problem of bad Decisions in the Choice of such Insurance Plans

Admittedly, many individuals may be expected to make a bad choice when offered an insurance plan that does not cover the newest medical technology later in life. Typically, fear of death will cause them to push the treating physician to try any treatment alternative regardless of cost provided it holds the promise of survival or even healing. At that point in time, they will quite likely regret not having opted for the more comprehensive plan that would give them access also to the very latest and most costly technology available.

But then, it needs to be recalled that freedom of choice always implies the risk of a regretted choice. The fact that consumers can choose a luxury car if they so wish implies that some of them will be dissatisfied after the purchase because the benefits are less than imagined and/or the user cost higher than envisaged. Getting rid of such a car is possible but entails substantial effort and financial sacrifice. Errors of this kind can certainly be avoided by having the government regulate the production of cars, presumably according to the philosophy of "one size fits all". The experience of the centrally planned economies has shown that such imposed homogeneity just about kills technological innovation.

One might argue that the choice of a health insurance plan involves a far more binding commitment than the choice of a car. However, there are choices in human life that involve even longer-term commitments, such as choice of a profession, of a marriage partner, and the decision to have one or several children. In all of these, people are known to make bad mistakes, and the cost of correcting them may be tremendous. Yet, few would argue that government should be called in to regulate these choices in an attempt to avoid costly errors.

Indeed, individuals who wish to regain access to the latest medical technology can do this at a high but not exorbitant cost. First, they can simply draw on their personal fortune to finance the extra cost associated with the particular treatment. Second, having profited from a reduced contribution for many years, they may have set aside at least part of the savings precisely for this event. Third, they can call on family members, friends, and charities to simply donate the money that is needed to cover the gap.

These considerations give rise to a third and final question: What is ethically recommendable about suppressing the choice of an insurance plan that offers lower premiums in return to restricted access to latest medical technology?

These questions shall not be answered here, as they clearly point beyond the domain of economic theory. Rather, it is up to the philosophers of ethics to address them. However, if no convincing answers should be forthcoming, the ethical basis of government-imposed rationing of health care services appears to be in serious doubt.

Global Budgets and Rationing

Rationing in Medicine:
Cost Containment versus Quality Improvement

Christof Szymkowiak

In Germany there is an ongoing discussion about future problems of the allocation of resources. All the experts discussing this topic have to acknowledge that the German health care system, which was designed 120 year ago, is still functioning, but nobody currently, knows how it still works and how long it will work.

However, it is undisputed that we will face two big problems affecting our health care system which, in the future, may even force us to change it dramatically by introducing some form of rationing of resources. The two main problems are:

- demographic change in society and multimorbity of the elderly
- technological progress, that will add new treatment options.

Both developments will put a major financial burden on the financing of our health care system unless we find ways to tackle the problem. There are right now two directions that we are following to deal with the development mentioned above:

- cost containment through budgeting procedures
- improving the quality of health care with the aim to use the given resources better and thus affording the possibility to save money in the long run to use for other problems.

1
Cost Containment

Everywhere we look we will find budgets. On governmental level, on the health care system level and on the private level. It is a way to deal with limited resources. In most cases, the resource involved is money, and the procedure one that we are all used to. Right now we are using sectoral budgets for the out-patient (ambulatory care), the in-patient (hospital care) sector and for prescriptions etc. Looking at the financial figures of 1999, we see that it has worked out fairly well again for this year. However, by using sectoral budgets for cost-containment, we have produced or intensified the problems of differentiating the boundaries, for example, between the in-patient and the out-patient sectors. Thereby creating problems for patients that need to cross these boundaries during their treatment and creating the problem of duplicating service in the different sectors.

In the last health care system act in Germany a global budget was imposed. The aim of the global budget was to get rid of the sectoral budgets that create many problems for patients crossing the boundaries during their treatment. In principle this idea is a good idea, because it implies that the health care insurance companies would be able to pay for services offered at the place of greatest efficiency. Boundaries between in-patient and out-patient sectors and even between professionals working in the different sectors would be reduced by the need to cooperate and subsequently there might be a chance to optimize the system.

Right now we are still in the phase of operationalizing a global budget. There are mayor obstacles to be overcome. One difficulty is to implement a global budget. In our country a lot of laws are made at the "Länder" (states) level and therefore individual "Länder" budgets and individual health insurance budgets are needed for 450 companies. But how do we control spending? By creating sub-budgets we would loose all the positive effects of abolishing sectoral budgets and most propably would create new problems.

A minor difficulty of a global budget is that there are different systems of re-imbursement for the out-patient (ambulatory care) and the in-patient sector (hospital care). To ensure that in-patient care does not eat up all the budget because of direct re-imbursement of the individual hospital by the insurance companies, a kind of budget is needed for the out-patient sector which allows re-imbursement only after a three-month time lag.

Therefore, at present, a global budget to solve the problems existing between different care sectors seems to be far away in the distant future.

2
Quality Improvement

A growing concern about the quality of care is the second driving force to change our health care system and also deals with our financial problems. First by questioning the appropriateness of services provided, second by putting our focus on outcomes of health care and third by strengthening the accountability of providers through internal and external quality assurance measures.

The methods of health technology assessment and the principles of evidence based medicine are used to improve the appropriateness of care. The use of treatment protocols and clinical practice guidelines is also on the increase.

Also of great importance is patient participation to define and measure outcome. Additionally we need to define strong and measurable outcome parameters. I will not go into further detail in this field, nor in the area of strengthening the accountability by quality assurance programmes and certification programmes.

These are the topics that are currently under discussion in the self governing bodies to improve the quality of the existing health care system. You may have noticed that I have not mentioned rationing yet. But it is of no doubt that by rationalization on a macro-level, the rationing of services is already taking place on the micro-level, on the level of physicians, i.e. that micro-level rationing already exists. For instance, simply by dealing in one way or the other with individual prescription budgets, or by treating patients at the beginning of a 3-month re-imbursement period differently from at the end of this period. This problem only applies to out-patient care. Depending upon whether or not it will harm the patient or withhold needed services this could by characterized as positive or negative rationing.

Therefore the rationalization of structures and processes might lead to rationing on the level of general practitioners unless ways to optimize processes and improve quality of care can be found. I mentioned the methods used before.

In my view, a global budget which has to be divided into sub-budgets, will not improve the current system and will not get rid of the problem of rationing that already exists. In order to make a global budget work, you must change much more. For example using the system of diagnosis related groups (DRG) spanning the in-patient and the out-patient sector and using the same re-imbursement system for all sectors.

There is a need to start a debate on rationing well ahead of time, while we are right now in a phase that is dominated by rationalization. If we don't start the debate, financial problems might overwhelm us. Furthermore, we should define the way we use the word rationing. Either in the way of the definition of rationing by Prof. Kliemt which might be best described as positive rationing, or we might even talk about negative rationing. Whether appropriateness of care belongs to the one or the other should be discussed later.

But we need something like a timetable or a work schedule:

- In my considered opinion, we should first try out all cost-containing measures that might stabilize the current system.
- Second we have to improve quality of care with the aim to prevent costly long-term effects.
- And third we have to start a debate *with* and *in* our society about rationing.

The self governed bodies can make suggestions regarding areas of rationing and will provide the evidence for these suggestions, but the decision whether our society should impose rationing or spend more money on health care should be made by all concerned.

III   Rationing, Ethics, and the Law

The Impact of the German Constitution on Rationing in Medicine

Jochen Taupitz

1
Introduction

Medical treatment requires – apart from non-materialistic resources such as time, affection and care[1] – a certain amount of materialistic and especially financial resources. In addition to materialistic resources such as donated organs being scarce, medical treatment is being rationed financially.

In order to discuss rationing in medicine, one must consider both the relationship between law and medicine as well as the extent to which financial resources influence them both. On the one hand one might fear that law has already entered too many aspects of medicine. On the other hand medicine can cause legal protection to be required. Due to this ambivalent relationship between medicine and law, the question arises as to what extent financial resources influence medicine and law[2] and whether legislation proves to be an accomplice to medicine in its battle against rationing.

2
Legal and Financial Aspects of Medical Treatment

Whereas legal, medical and financial experts acknowledge the fact that there is a lack of financial resources in the German health system, their points of view differ considerably in regard to the effect which is caused by the lack of resources. From an economist's point of view, rationing causes a *statistical* risk of not being treated adequately[3] whereas both doctor and lawyer have to deal with the medical treatment history of the *"real" individual patient:* The *doctor's* interest is focused on the patient's physical condition as well as on the question whether or not his patient can be treated successfully.[4] *Lawyer* and *judge* will examine the doctor's performance in an individual case and from there the possibility and need of confronting him with liability claims.

---

[1]   See Fuchs, Kostendämpfung und ärztlicher Standard – Verantwortlichkeit und Prinzipien der Ressourcenverteilung, MedR 1993, p 323.

[2]   Instructive to this problem is the discussion between Krämer, Medizin muss rationiert werden (medicine must be rationed), MedR 1996, p 1; Bossman, Rationierung medizinischer Leistungen (rationing medical services), MedR 1996, p 456.

[3]   Krämer, (as in note no. 2), p 5.

[4]   Fuchs, Allokationsprobleme bei knappen Ressourcen, in: Nagel/Fuchs (ed), Soziale Gerechtigkeit im Gesundheitswesen, 1993, pp 6, 14.

Danger arises as soon as both medicine and law are *dictated* by financial aspects. If the law primarily aims at calling forth *financially* effective behaviour in people, this will surely have an impact both on patients as well as on physicians.[5] Compared to the situation in the United States, German jurisdiction has so far not been based on the so called Economic Analysis of Law[6] which gives financial effectiveness a great influence on the legal system. Nevertheless financial aspects are of importance as far as legislation is being influenced by the idea of economic effectiveness or as far as it allows an interpretation under a financial point of view.[7]

I would now like to draw the focus of attention on the dimensions of constitutional law. This point of view is of particular importance since Parliament as the legislative body, acting often motivated by daily politics, is bound to constitutional regulations itself. Therefore, constitutional regulations lead to a more long-term perspective – despite all uncertainties of interpretation.

In order to answer the question whether constitutional rights might serve in the battle against rationing one must distinguish between the right to a specific health service, the right to a non-discriminatory distribution of health services and the right to receive appropriate information as a patient.

3
On the Existence of a Constitutional Right to a Specific Health Service

The question whether or not the German Constitution grants the right to a specific health service is of particular importance for the possibility of setting constitutional limits to rationing in medicine. If such a constitutional right does in fact exist, it will draw a line against too many rationalising measures.

The German Constitution grants fundamental rights. These rights, however, must be mainly understood as protection against undue interventions by the state; in general they do not entitle an individual to claim specific services or acts.[8] Correspondingly, the Federal Constitutional Court has decided that due to the German Constitution the state is only obliged to provide for a health care system which is not totally insufficient or inappropriate, but that the constitution does not open a

---

5   Compare Hoppe's warning, Hoppe, Rhein. Ärztebl. 1998, p 15: "Siegeszug der Ökonomie gefährdet Arzt-Patienten-Verhältnis" ("The victory of rationing endangers the relationship between the doctor and his patient"); against a discussion solely under financial aspects see Roellecke, Was sind uns die Parteien wert? ("How much are the parties worth to us?"), in: Engel, Morlok (ed), Öffentliches Recht als ein Gegenstand ökonomischer Forschung, 1998, pp 61, 65.

6   Taupitz, Ökonomische Analyse und Haftungsrecht – eine Zwischenbilanz, AcP 196 (1996), pp 114, 128, 155.

7   Taupitz, Ressourcenknappheit in der Medizin – Hilfestellung durch das Grundgesetz?, in: Wolter, Riedel, Taupitz (ed), Einwirkungen der Grundrechte auf das Zivilrecht, Öffentliche Recht und Strafrecht, 1999, pp 113, 115.

8   Isensee, in: Handbuch des Staatsrechts, vol. V, 1992, § 111 marginal notes pp 93–95.

claim of a citizen against the statutory health insurance system for the provision and the guarantee of specific health services[9]. Therefore, the legislator was allowed even to establish the principle of economising (Wirtschaftlichkeitsgebot, § 12 SGB V) and by doing so he was allowed to limit the claims and rights of the citizens against the statutory health insurance system.[10] One must consider that this also concerns the treatment of patients in direct mortal danger although life protection is one of the main goals of the constitution. If this was not true, the responsible persons within the health system would have to concentrate the available funds primarily on the intensive care units in order to help any patient in peril of his life in preference to all persons who are not in direct mortal danger; and they would have to do so "at all costs" and even if there was only the slightest chance for the patient to survive or to prolong his life for a minimum period of time – an obligation which has not been demanded by anyone, so far, and which cannot be demanded reasonably.

Furthermore, it is of importance that the conclusion to deny a constitutional right to specific health services does not only concern the question of creating the availability of health services but also the question of access to those health services which are already on the market. Therefore a decision to refuse a certain therapy or operation because it is too expensive to be financed by the statutory health insurance system[11] would not contradict the German Constitution.

4
The Distribution of Health Services

Whereas the patient is denied a right to specific health services, he is granted a constitutional right to a non-discriminatory *distribution* of health services. However, the fair distribution of health services which are already on the market entitles a patient to "his share" of the available services. Consequently, a right to specific health services can arise after all if they are available to other patients under the same conditions. Yet this kind of specific right has to be understood as a result of a fair distribution and can therefore only reach as far as the already existing resources allow; an independent right to specific health services as discussed above under 3 does not exist.

The right to a non-discriminatory distribution of health services is due to the fact that only those criteria of distribution are permitted which offer – in principle – all

---

[9] BVerfG, MedR 1997, p 318.
[10] Taupitz (as in note no. 7), p 120.
[11] See Höfling, Rationierung von Gesundheitsleistungen im grundrechtsgeprägten Sozialstaat, in: Feuerstein/Kuhlmann (ed), Rationierung im Gesundheitswesen, 1998, pp 143, 148; Jarass, in: Jarass, Pieroth, GG, 3rd edition 1995, Art 2, marginal note 49a; Murswiek, in: Sachs, GG, 1996, Art. 2 marginal note 225; Künschner, Wirtschaftlicher Behandlungsverzicht und Patientenauswahl, 1992, p 255; Schreiber, Rechtliche Kriterien der Verteilungsgerechtigkeit im Sozialstaat, in: Nagel, Fuchs (ed), Soziale Gerechtigkeit (as in note no. 4), p 302.

persons affected the same chances.[12] In other words, the criteria of distribution must be "blind to status", which means that they should neither openly nor latently lead to a preferential treatment or non treatment of certain social or religious groups or to a selection regarding sex.[13]

Therefore, the German Constitution prohibits any consideration of social status as it is – for example – discussed in the United States.[14] Not only is it almost impossible to decide whether a mother of three children has a higher social value than a young business man, but, even more important, the constitutional principle of *equality* of human life *prohibits* the allocation of health services on such a basis. The decision to exclude recipients of welfare services from certain medical services (for example kidney transplantation) – as it is partly accepted in the United States[15] – would contravene the German Constitution.

For similar reasons, fixed age limits for certain kinds of treatment are not compatible with the German Constitution as they inevitably lead to a discrimination of very old or very young people.[16] Therefore, we could not follow the custom which has been practised in Great Britain for a long period of time where – in principle – no dialysis was offered to patients older than 60 or 65 years of age.[17] From the German point of view, age limits are permitted only if they correspond to medical criteria, for example regarding certain risks.[18] The Federal Court of Justice for instance, considered it to be reasonable that the availability of *amniocentesis* for the early diagnosis of Morbus Down is bound – in case of scarce resources – to a certain age of the pregnant women because the risk of Morbus Down is considerably higher from the age of 35 years onwards.[19]

---

[12] Compare with V. Schmidt, Verteilungsgerechtigkeit in der Transplantationsmedizin: Was kann die Soziologie beitragen?, Ethik in der Medizin 1998, pp 5, 9; Kirchhof, FAZ No. 125 from June 2nd 1998, p 11; see further to the rule of medical ethics that the physician is not allowed to distinguish between patients in regard to their religion, nationality, race, political privilege or social stand, Narr, Hess, Schirmer, Ärztliches Berufsrecht, 2nd edition 1997, marginal note B 114.

[13] This is clearly expressed in Art. 3 of the German Constitution.

[14] See Alexander, They Decide Who Lives, Who Dies, Life No. 53 of Nov 9th 1962, p 102; Giles, Medical Ethics, 1983, p 184; Beauchamp, Childress, Principles of Biomedical Ethics, 4th edition, 1994, p 384.

[15] Compare Fuchs (as in note no. 4), p 10; rejecting this quite rightly Giesen, Ethische und rechtliche Probleme am Ende des Lebens, JZ 1990, pp 929, 942.

[16] For complete detail see Harris, Der Wert des Lebens: eine Einführung in die medizinische Ethik, 1995, p 134; see further Oberender, in: Nagel, Fuchs (ed), Rationalisierung und Rationing im deutschen Gesundheitswesen, 1998, pp 10, 21.

[17] Giving statistics for Germany and other countries Prottas, Segal, Sapolsky, Cross-National Differences in Dialysis, Health Care Financing Review 1983, 91, p 97; see further Uhlenbruck, Rechtliche Grenzen einer Rationierung in der Medizin, MedR 1995, pp 427, 430; Fuchs (as in note no. 4), pp 6, 10; the same, Probleme der Makro- und Mikroallokation, in: Mohr, Schubert (ed), Ethik der Gesundheitsökonomie, 1992, p 67; Luf, Verteilungsgerechtigkeit im Bereich der modernen Medizin – Rechtsethische Überlegungen, RdM 1997, p 99.

[18] Harris (as in note no. 16), p 164.

[19] BGH NJW 1987, p 2923.

Medical criteria of treatment or non treatment are generally accepted by the law which implicitly means that criteria of distribution do exist. As a result the law referring to the distribution of scarce resources returns a great deal of the responsibility of decision-making to the medical profession and accepts various possible solutions as being equally fair or just. This does not mean an abdication of responsibility but the *distribution* of competences between different disciplines and – as a consequence – the distribution of responsibilities.[20]

All in all, the dominant principle both in medicine and in our legal system must always be the principle of commensurability (Verhältnismäßigkeitsgrundsatz) which combines – in case of scarce resources – the protection of the individual with the principle of equality.[21]

5
Civil Liability

This leads us to the question what effect the return of responsibility of decision-making to the medical profession has on the civil liability of a physician. First of all, there is the rule of "impossibilium nulla est obligatio" – the law does not oblige anyone to do something that is not possible. However, defining what is possible and what is impossible is not only a problem of the specific situation – but it is also a problem of planning and of considering the future. In terms of civil liability we call this phenomenon the problem of "Organisationsverschulden" – the liability for mis-organising. The physician is obliged to organise his sphere in a way that the scarce resources are distributed according to the principle of commensurability. Although it is true that the physician should always consider his next patient to be the most important one, he has to – while treating the present patient – take into account the needs of the next patient as well as of other future patients.

6
The Distribution of Scarce Resources and the Autonomy of Patients

This leads to a third aspect of possible constitutional rights regarding rationing in medicine and scarce resources. In addition to guaranteeing a fair distribution of health services, the German Constitution protects the autonomy of patients.[22] In my opinion this aspect will become even more important in the future.

---

[20] Taupitz (as in note no. 7), p 126.

[21] On the principle of commensurability regarding medical treatment see Laufs, Arztrecht, 5th edition, 1993, marginal note 491.

[22] On the constitutional foundation of the patient's autonomy and informed consent see Glatz, Der Arzt zwischen Beratung und Aufklärung, 1998, p 228; Taupitz, Empfehlen sich zivilrechtliche Regelungen zur Absicherung der Patientenautonomie am Ende des Lebens?, Gutachten A zum 63. Deutschen Juristentag, 2000, p A 12.

The German jurisprudence has often decided that there is no need to inform the patient about the fact that there are other hospitals which provide a higher level of competence, equipment and so on.[23] In contrast to this I believe that if – for financial reasons – there is an increasing distinction in health services concerning the supply on either a maximum, a normal or a minimum level, this enlargement of the "medical corridor" must result in a stronger emphasis on the aspect of autonomy and self-determination on the part of the patient affected.[24] The patient must be enabled – on the basis of appropriate information – to decide for himself whether he wishes to be treated – if necessary at his own expenses – by another doctor or in another hospital where "his" requirements are satisfied.[25] Only with this reservation (informing the patient in advance), one can tolerate that the patient must accept insufficient capacities for particular treatments without having a right to compensation, as it has been decided by the courts.[26] Thus, the patient must be informed about the fact that an operation which is not immediately necessary but reasonable[27] cannot be done in the near future because of scarce resources. The information should enable him to look for another institution where an operation is possible without delay.[28] Not only the principle of methodical honesty but particularly the professional liability of doctors and the need for confidence in the patient-physician relationship call for the *separation* and *transparency* of medical and economic reasons.[29]

Therefore, from the patient's point of view and due to the patient's autonomy, *complete information* is required, in other words, we should come to an *open rationing*.[30] This does not mean a duty to explain any possible financial aspect,[31] but the physician's duty to inform the patient about the fact that a treatment is being refused solely because of the high costs although the treatment is necessary or at least reasonable from the medical point of view. However, the other side of this development will be that the responsibility of distribution of scarce resources will increasingly be shifted towards the patient. Once again, this shows that the protection provided by constitutional rights as far as it is based on the responsibility of

---

23 For quotations see Steffen, Dressler, Arzthaftungsrecht – Neue Entwicklungslinien der BGH-Rechtsprechung, 7th edition 1997, p 134.

24 Rightly so Hart, Rechtliche Grenzen der "Ökonomisierung", MedR 1996, pp 60, 69.

25 About the duty to inform the patient about the possibility that better diagnosis and better treatment might be available elsewhere, see also Makiol, Begründen eingeschränkte Leistungspflichten der gesetzlichen Krankenversicherung neue Aufklärungspflichten des Arztes?, in: Arbeitsgemeinschaft Rechtsanwälte im Medizinrecht e.V. (ed), Die Budgetierung im Gesundheitswesen, 1997, p 105; further Hübner, NJW 1989, pp 5, 7 – see also on what the German health ministers agreed upon in a conference in 1996, MedR 1997, p 460; further Katzenmeier, Qualität im Gesundheitswesen, MedR 1997, p 498.

26 Rumler-Detzel, Budgetierung – Rationalisierung – Rationierung, VersR 1998, pp 546, 548.

27 Compare OLG Köln, VersR 1993, p 52.

28 Taupitz, (as in note no. 7), p 132.

29 Hart, (as in note no. 24), p 70.

30 See Fuchs, Was heißt hier Rationierung?, in: Nagel, Fuchs (ed), Rationalisierung (as in note no. 16), pp 42, 44.

31 For this see for example Glatz (as in note no. 22), pp 284, 327.

decision-making and on the autonomy of the person protected, can also include a burden, albeit the fundamental rights are not converted to fundamental duties.

7
Conclusion

The impact which scarce resources in general and financial aspects in particular have upon medical treatment cannot be ignored by law. In order to answer the question whether constitutional rights might serve in the battle against rationing one must distinguish between the right to a specific health service, the right to a non-discriminatory distribution of health services and the right to receive appropriate information as a patient.

While the patient does not have a constitutional right to specific and sometimes very expensive health services, he does have a constitutional right to a non-discriminatory distribution of health services. That means that a right to specific health services can arise as a consequence to a non-discriminatory distribution; in other words this right only exists in case specific health services are available for other patients under the same conditions. Last but not least, the patient has a constitutional right to be given appropriate information, which also embraces financial aspects of treatment or non-treatment.

Conclusion

Rationing Yes, Politics No. For a Right-based Approach in Rationing Medical Goods*

Michael Baurmann

1
Basic Assumptions and Goals of the Discussion

I presuppose, firstly, that medical resources are limited and that not every need for medical treatment can be satisfied. Secondly, I presuppose that we do not want to give up a publicly funded health system altogether. However, I will not discuss the reasons in favour of a publicly funded health system here. I simply want to say that a preference for such a health system does not in my opinion exclude the possibility of an additional provision by private insurances. Neither will I make any assumptions with regard to the size of the budget for a publicly funded health system but I think that it will include at a minimum level what can be called a "basic coverage".

If these two presuppositions hold true we then have to answer the question of allocation: according to which criteria should the limited medical resources which are supplied by the state be distributed among those requiring treatment? There seem to be two principal options in answering this question: *equality* or *maximisation*. Their implications with regard to the distribution of vital goods can be illustrated by an example. Imagine that a limited number of life-boats has to be allocated on a ship. According to the principle of equality the boats should be distributed in a way that gives every passenger an *equal chance of survival*. If the aim is maximisation the distribution of boats should try instead to *maximise the survival rate* of the passengers. The distribution of the boats on the various decks can differ significantly in both cases.

If we prefer an allocation of – publicly funded – medical goods according to a principle of equality this would mean in analogy to the distribution of life-boats that everyone should have a right to the same quality of medical treatment, that every ill person has an equal chance to get his illness cured or alleviated. The alternative would be an allocation of these scarce medical goods according to a principle of maximisation – similar to the maximisation of the survival rate of passengers on a ship. This principle can be applied on the macro level of political decisions as well as on the meso and micro level of decisions by hospitals or doctors. It would imply, for example, that on the level of macro-allocation hospitals are only built in areas with a high density of population or on a level of micro-allocation that doctors make a deliberate selection among possible recipients of medical treatment and save medical resources for those who have the best prospects. In this case not

---

* Translation by Margaret Birbeck. I thank Hartmut Kliemt for his indispensable comments and hints.

everyone would have a right to be given the same medical attendance but rather medical treatment would be distributed according to some discriminating criteria. At the margin each unit of money spent on health care would have to yield the same return in terms of cured individuals or lives saved (presumably adjusted by some quality index or other).

Prima facie there seem to be good arguments in favour of rationing restricted medical goods by a rule of maximisation. This strategy in general provides the opportunity to exploit limited resources optimally by using them deliberately in spheres where they have the highest degree of effectiveness. Given that suitable criteria are available – for example maximising life expectancy or "quality-adjusted life years" ("qalys") – the efficiency of a health system will be enhanced significantly if its resources are distributed accordingly. And would such an improvement of efficiency not be in the interest of all concerned? Would it not be the case that a health system that maximises life expectancy or qalys on a general level would also maximise the life expectancy or qalys of every individual? And should not everyone therefore prefer such a health system to a system which distributes its resources without any maximising choices?

In the following I will contradict these seemingly suggestive arguments by putting forward some considerations *against* maximisation and *pro* equality. Or to put it in a slightly different way: I will reason against a consequentialist approach in rationing medical goods and will argue instead for a right-based approach. It should be remembered though that my considerations refer only to a publicly funded health system. They cannot be simply transferred to questions which are connected with private health insurances (cf. Breyer and Kliemt 1994; Kliemt 1995; 1996). And I should say from the outset that my arguments are not applicable either to emergency situations where the problem of "triage" occurs (cf. on this W. Lübbe in this volume). My arguments are directed solely to the question how we should design institutions which have to cope with the distribution of limited medical goods in normal everyday practice.

I will discuss the problem of the allocation of scarce medical resources by way of a digression. I will first take a look at the way in which we regulate the distribution of *other* elementary goods. It may seem that here I can find quick and strong support for my assertion concerning the superiority of a right-based approach also in the case of medical care. It appears to be evident that we in general prefer a framework of rights and equality when distributing vital goods instead of a consequentialist principle of efficiency and maximisation.

2
Taking Maximisation Seriously

If we look at the usual justification of the predominance of right-based theories we find that in the context of *civil rights* it is often argued that maximisation and efficiency as utilitarian principles are collectivistic and show disregard for individual interests. If we apply these principles, it is said, public welfare will override individual welfare. A central embarrassment for such consequentialist or goal-based theories is, as for example John L. Mackie puts it, "that they not merely allow but positively require, in certain circumstances, that the well-being of one individual should be sacrificed ... for the well-being of others." (Mackie 1978, p 352).

Rights, on the other hand, are seen as protecting the interests of the individual against collective welfare. An order of rights therefore "is *not* saddled with the embarrassing presumption that one person's well-being can be simply replaced by that of another" (Mackie 1978, p 359). Or to put it in the well-known words of another prominent advocate of rights, Ronald Dworkin, rights are *trumps* in the hand of the individual against the claims of the community (Dworkin 1978).

Because civil rights are supposed to be clearly recognizable as safeguarding the individual, this line of reasoning ends with the conclusion that from an individualistic point of view an order of rights is by far preferable to an order of utilitarian maximisation. It would appear to be obvious that a right-based system protects individual interests far better than any other institution.

Closer inspection reveals, however, that this line of argument is, unfortunately, too simple and is missing an important dimension. In fact, even from a strictly individualistic point of view there are good prima facie reasons for adopting a utilitarian principle of maximisation – especially when we are dealing with goods of high value such as are related to civil rights. The alternative between efficiency-based institutions and right-based institutions is not a simple alternative between giving priority to individual interests or giving priority to collective interests. Even under the premise of an individualistic position the superiority of a right-based allocation of goods is not at all evident.

The frequent self-confident appeal to ration medical goods according to a principle of maximisation is thus an indicator of a problem which in my opinion seems to be underestimated in the context of the general discussion on civil rights. Obviously not all advocates of medical rationing by maximisation are anti-liberal "collectivists". On the contrary they assume that such a health system would be in the interest of all of us individually. It follows that we have to take maximisation more seriously – especially if we want to present sound arguments *against* it!

But *why* are there good prima facie reasons for a principle of utilitarian maximisation from an individualistic point of view? These reasons become clear when we place ourselves in an *ex-ante-situation* where we have to choose between different rules for the future distribution of vital goods. If we weigh up our interests in such an ex-ante-situation, it seems to be in the best interest of *all of us* to choose a rule of maximisation instead of a right-based order. The fundamental reason for this is that ex-ante the chance of becoming the beneficiary of a rule of maximisation is greater than of becoming its victim. And this also applies in respect to those basic goods which are candidates for the protection by civil rights.

According to a rule of maximisation the distribution of basic goods such as personal freedom, freedom of speech, health, physical integrity or protection against arbitrary punishment would only then deviate from equality as it is incorporated in an order of civil rights if this enhanced the overall welfare. But this means that *ex-ante* everyone would benefit from such a maximising device because all persons concerned would improve their individual chances with regard to their future personal share of this welfare. Hence it appears to be an obvious and perfectly rational choice for everyone to favour a principle of maximisation and not an order of rights.

This decision does, of course, imply an acceptance of a restriction of civil liberties in situations in which the overall benefit of such measures would surpass their disadvantages. This might be any of the following cases. The execution of a man for a crime he did not commit if several other lives were saved by the deterrent effect. The imprisonment of innocent members of the family of a dangerous criminal if this prevented him from committing serious crimes. The torture of a suspect in order to extract information on the location of a hidden bomb. The expropriation of a landowner if this improved the situation of a great number of other people. The restriction of the freedom of speech whenever the danger of civil riots exists. And last but not least, the use of someone as an organ bank if this could save the lives of several other people (cf. Harris 1980). To me it seems indisputable that there are, in fact, situations in which such intrusions in the elementary interests of certain individuals would indeed be the welfare-maximising choice.

As is well-known it is crucial to Rawls' theory that such ex-ante decisions behind a veil of ignorance would, in contrary, *not* be in favour of utilitarian and consequentialist principles but in favour of a regime of rights. As I see it, he puts forward mainly two arguments to refute considerations like the above. His first argument claims that someone who is risk-averse would prefer a future situation in which his basic interests are secured by rights in all events against being sacrificed for the interests of others (Rawls 1971, ch. 3, § 28). But this argument is not sound. Rawls does not take into account the important fact that an individual can rationally expect to advance exactly these basic interests by a maximising rule: if, for example, one person is sacrificed so that three others can survive (by the transplantation of his organs or by his punishment as an innocent man), then one would increase one's chances of survival ex-ante if one opted for a rule of maximisation and *not* for an unconditional right to live.

The same holds true for other goods which are protected by civil rights. There are always situations imaginable in which I can benefit from the violation of the rights of others to promote for myself exactly the kind of interests which are the subject of these rights. One cannot, as Rawls does, only take cases into account in which rights may be violated in favour of aggregated inferior benefits.

Rawls' second argument hints at the problems which would probably emerge if we tried to execute a principle of maximisation in practice (Rawls 1971, ch. 3, § 29). Rawls is right in claiming that we should only opt for principles which can be realised without making excessive demands on people and thereby endangering the stability of society. We should therefore only consent to decisions in ex-ante situations which everyone of us can also keep ex-post. This is an important argument and I will come back to it presently. Unfortunately Rawls' own rejection of a rule of maximisation on the grounds of this adequate claim is hardly acceptable. Rawls argues that under unfavourable conditions this rule would demand "unbearable" sacrifices from some people in favour of the well-being of others. If this ex-post result comes about we cannot expect the "losers" to observe an ex-ante agreement any longer. Rawls goes on by saying that this danger could be avoided if a system of rights was established because then nobody would run the risk of a violation of his own basic interests for the benefit of others.

But this is only half the truth. The argument has to be elaborated on further. The situations under a rule of maximisation and under a right-based system are more symmetrical than Rawls suggests. It is not correct to state that in the first case some people who are the "losers" have to sacrifice basic interests for the sake of the "winners", whereas in the second case no one will run the risk of becoming a loser. If, for example, under a rule of maximisation one person had to give his life as an organ-donor for the life of three other persons, his life would indeed be spared under a rule of rights – but it should not be overlooked that the price for *his* right is to be paid by the *other* three persons who now have to give their lives for the life of the potential donor! So likewise, in a right-based system there are of necessity "winners" and "losers". And at first glance it is not at all evident that the three victims in our example have more reason to accept their fate than the organ-donor who is compelled to give his organs in the first place.

The protection of rights *always* has the price of the potential gains which could be earned by their violation. It is not true that these costs in most cases are insignificant for those who have to bear them (this is perfectly clear in the "trolley-case": cf. Rakowski 1993; Thomson 1985). In order to make sense of Rawls' assumption that there is a fundamental problem connected with the practical implementation of a rule of maximisation which would not emerge in the case of a right-based system we have to take a closer look at the problem.

To sum up we can say that up to now we have heard no convincing argument why – from an ex-ante point of view – a right-based system of equal distribution would be preferable to a rule of maximisation as a device for a discriminating distribution of vital goods. And this result does not presuppose any bias towards some sort of "collectivistic" reasoning where individual interests are principally subordinate to the common welfare. The "embarrassment" for consequentialist theories i.e. that they could require the sacrifice of individual well-being to the interests of the majority poses no threat to individuals if it is duly recognised that the beneficiaries of such sacrifices are also individuals and their interests. It seems to be that we are therefore forced to acknowledge the fact that rights do not *per se* guarantee the best possible outcome for each individual.

3
Why Rights?

Nevertheless we have to admit that it is very unlikely that anybody would derive strong motives from these facts to abolish our right-based institutions in the area of civil liberties. Because of this we should be cautious in the case of the distribution of medical goods, too. The fact that there seem to be good ex-ante reasons for allocating limited medical goods according to a maximising rule should perhaps not be overrated. If there are sufficient similarities with the case of civil rights and the refusal of a rule of maximisation turns out to be well-founded here we maybe have good reasons to establish a right-based regime as well in the field of health care.

To prove this we now have to turn to the question *why* we do not apparently consider our ex-ante interests important enough to alter our preference for civil rights and replace them by some kind of efficiency-based institutions. My thesis is that: *if* we are in an ex-ante situation and *if* a rule of maximisation would improve our expectations in contrast to a rule of rights, we would only decide in favour of this option on condition that it could be guaranteed that

1. a rule of maximisation would be defined and applied in a *neutral* and *impartial* way, and that
2. we could trust in a *mechanism of commitment* which would bind all participants to a rule of maximisation ex-post as well.

I think that as rational actors we are not against maximising per se. But I think we are right to opt against maximisation in many cases because we cannot rationally expect a neutral and impartial institutionalisation and execution of a rule of maximisation and also because there is no mechanism of commitment efficient enough to prevent people from breaking their contracts if their vital interests are at stake. Both doubts are directly connected with the fact that maximisation only is feasible as a *political enterprise* in the fields which are of interest here. Its aims can only be realised by *collective decisions* on a bundle of questions. If, for example, I have the right to live, questions concerning my life and death are not subject to collective decisions. In the case of unrestricted maximisation, conditions under which I am allowed to live and under which I am forced to die *have to be* legally subject to collective decisions.

Seen from this point of view we can now recognise a fundamental difference between a system of maximisation and a system of rights which has not yet been taken into account: Rights are instruments to *limit* the domain of politics in principle and to *reduce* the legal range of collective decisions. The establishment of a rule of maximisation is on the contrary inevitably connected with *political empowerment*. Rights embody a claim to political *omission* and *limitation* whereas rules of maximisation embody a claim to political *activity* and therefore to an *enlargement* of political power.

But *why* should we hesitate to impose upon politics the duty of maximisation in the sphere which is now protected by civil rights? Why should we doubt that politics would apply a rule of maximisation in a way that suits the ex-ante interests of the citizens and expect instead that politics will necessarily or very probably come into conflict with the demand for impartiality and commitment to former decisions?

To answer these questions we do *not* need to presuppose a worst-case scenario. It would not be difficult to give reasons against entrusting a rule of maximisation to an autocratic regime. But the decisive point can be made already in the case of democratic politics under the rule of law. We have to realise that there are at least three kinds of crucial decisions relevant in the course of establishing and practising a system of maximisation. We can call them "decisions on operationalisation", "decisions on implementation" and "decisions on application". Decisions on operationalisation are necessary to transform the principle of maximisation into a manageable rule as a guideline for practice. Decisions on implementation are necessary to establish institutions and rules of procedure for the everyday application of a rule of maximisation. And decisions on application are necessary to determine for concrete cases the consequences of a rule of maximisation.

The problem with this kind of decisions is that their very nature makes them susceptible to arbitrary influences. To operationalise a rule of maximisation we are not in possession of objective criteria which would guarantee an optimal result for a distribution of goods, burdens, and services. There are no intersubjectively valid standards available to judge the neutrality of such criteria. A large number of alternatives also exist for an institutional and procedural implementation of a rule of maximisation. It is not evident which of them serves the aim of predictability and neutrality in the application of a rule of maximisation best. And last but not least an application of rules which should produce efficient results is in particular tempting for "teleological" reasoning by which a clever interpreter of a rule can easily override its literal meaning by referring to its true "aim".

Therefore, there is ample room for *discretion* in the case of decisions on operationalisation as well as in the case of decisions on implementation and application. And it is a priori *improbable* that in a democracy the neutrality and impartiality of these decisions can be guaranteed.

There are two main reasons for this sceptical assessment:

The first reason is that common ex-ante interests in establishing a rule of maximisation depend on the fact that the participants do not yet know whether they will belong to the winners or losers of this rule. However, that does not prevent them from also having a vital ex-ante interest *not* to belong to the losers in the future but to the winners. *And* they have – at least to some extent – ex-ante knowledge how to operationalise, implement and apply a rule of maximisation so that *they* will not belong to the losers but to the winners – for example in regard to exclusion clauses which restrict the applicability of a general rule. It follows that everyone has ex-ante a strong incentive to form a majority coalition to influence democratic decisions of operationalisation and implementation such as to privilege members of his own group and to *exclude* them from the group of potential losers of a rule of maximisation.

The second reason is that the interests of the participants will *change* ex-post. Common ex-ante interests with regard to a rule of maximisation depend on common risks. In the course of time risks will change, probabilities become calculable, some risks will become reality, others not. The participants will increasingly gain knowledge whether they will join the losers or the winners of a rule of maximisation. Accordingly their evaluation of such a rule will change. So generally there will also be strong incentives ex-post for everyone to form a majority coalition to influence the operationalisation, implementation and application of a rule of maximisation in their own particular interests. These incentives will work against any commitment in favour of an ex-ante agreement.

The room for discretion inevitably allowed by any rule of maximisation and the veil of the rhetorics of common welfare will allow for far-reaching adjustments to a rule of maximisation in the course of its establishment and execution. A path of development will start which will transform the original rule of maximisation to a pure rule of redistribution in the interest of the ruling majorities. In the cases where basic goods are involved, the dynamics will accelerate because of the danger of irreversible damages (cf. on the process of politicisation in particular de Jasay 1991).

These prospects will produce a preference for right-based institutions if the losses one has to fear as a member of a minority outweigh the benefits one can hope for as a member of a majority. This is likely to happen because a majority will have no reason to give up any small advantage even at the expense of a large disadvantage of the minority. Under this condition a constitutional system of rights which *as a matter of principle* forbids maximisation resp. redistribution by sub-constitutional collective decisions makes everyone better off. This would be true ex-ante and could also be true for most of the people ex-post – given a democracy in which majorities will cycle with certain probabilities (cf. Buchanan/Congleton 1998).

The scales would tip even more to an order of rights if one takes into account the cost of investments in the process of political decision-making which have to be made to preserve one's chances in the political fight for redistribution. Generally political power would gain much more weight and the incentives to participate in the struggle for influential political positions would increase considerably (cf. Buchanan/Congleton 1998). If one argues in favour of the plausibility of a rule of maximisation on the grounds of ex-ante interests one should not forget ex-post interests which lead to the instability and politicisation of such a rule.

If these considerations are well-grounded the idea of rights is not to realize the best possible world. The idea is to give up the aim to strive for the best possible world *by political decisions*. To opt for right-based institutions would amount to renouncing the potential gains which can be realized by a rule of maximisation.

4
Right-based Rationing

What are the consequences of all this for the problem of rationing limited medical resources which are supplied by public funding?

First of all: private goods of fundamental importance are at stake in this case, too. This means that the incentives to become a winner and not a loser will be at least as urgent as in the case of the vital goods which are protected by civil rights. There is an important difference, however: the goods which are at stake in the context of health care cannot be guaranteed by the state by *omitting* certain acts but only by *active performance*. Therefore if one wants to establish rights in this area those rights would be *claim rights* and not the *negative rights* of the classical liberal constitution.

But in one essential aspect – which is of special importance here – there is a decisive similarity between claim rights and negative rights. Claim rights as well as negative rights *limit* the range of collective decision effectively. If one has a claim right to a certain good then it is not the object of collective decision whether one should receive the good or not.

Thus we face the same fundamental alternative as in the case of civil liberties: we can either organise the allocation of scarce medical goods by right-based institutions to ensure equality of distribution or by efficiency-based institutions which would distribute medical goods by some rule of maximisation. In the case of right-based allocation everyone would have a right to the same quality of medical treatment; in the case of an efficiency-based allocation the aim would be to maximise the probability of success, the rate of survival or "qalys".

We can now argue by analogy to the case of civil rights. Ex-ante there seem to be convincing reasons for everyone to opt for an efficiency-based institution. For everyone the chances of good health, survival or qalys would be maximised. But as in the case of other basic goods a choice of a rule of maximisation would only be imperative if one could rely on the impartial and neutral establishment and execution of such a rule – and if we have good reason for mistrust in other cases we should also be suspicious in the present one.

In the case of maximising medical goods nobody wants to become a loser either and so will have incentives to invest in political decision-making to prevent a bad lot. Everybody will prefer ex-ante a rule of maximisation which is operationalised and implemented in a way that he is excluded a priori from the potential group of losers. Everybody will try to change a rule of maximisation ex-post to join the group of winners. The votes of all these persons will be on the market and available to political entrepreneurs who offer themselves as agents of special interest-groups.

Therefore we must expect similar tendencies to politicise a rule of maximisation in the field of medical goods and to transform this rule in a game of pure re-distribution in favour of the ruling majorities. Taking into account the elementary importance of the goods at stake the dynamics against neutrality and impartiality and for an erosion of commitments to former agreements should be even more forceful. The slippery slope could be particularly steep.

Taking all aspects into account it seems to me that if we have good reasons for establishing an order of civil rights we also have good reasons for establishing an order of rights in the field of public health.

Let me finally consider very briefly what it could mean to establish a right-based allocation of limited medical resources. What could it mean to have the same right to medical treatment if unrestricted medical treatment is not available? Obviously it cannot mean that everybody has a right to the *best* treatment. But it could mean that everybody has an equal right to treatment of the *same quality*.

What this principle entails is fairly clear with regard to persons who suffer the same kind of illness. It is much less clear with regard to persons who suffer *different* kinds of illnesses. How can we measure whether the treatment of an influenza is of the same quality as the treatment of some type of cancer? But it does not seem entirely hopeless to make sense of the idea that different forms of medical treatment can have the same quality. One step in this direction would be to form classes of illnesses where they are differentiated, for example, according to their degree of danger, their typical impairment of life-quality or their consequences in the case of non-treatment. This would extend the sets of illnesses to which the criteria of equal treatment could be applied more or less straightforwardly. In a second step one can then try to compare the consequences for the different classes of illnesses if we have to make certain curtailments on an optimal treatment. Even if we cannot compare the quality of treatment for influenza with the quality of treatment for cancer directly we can perhaps do so with regard to the consequences it would have in both cases if some forms of possible treatment were *not* provided.

But there is another possibility to realise the idea of equal rights to medical treatment which perhaps sounds more convincing. According to this proposal a publicly funded health system would – within the limits of the given restrictions – offer different packages of medical treatment. These packages may differ consider-ably in the combination of medical services they offer. Some may put their main emphasis on a basic coverage for all types of illness whereas others may concentrate on an extensive treatment of severe diseases. Every citizen would obtain the right to choose one of those packages. In this way we would get rid of the difficult question what exactly is meant by the equal treatment of different diseases. We would interpret equal rights to medical treatment as equal rights to choose between different offers of medical treatment according to individual preferences.

I think that there are more and perhaps much better possibilities to realise the idea of an equal right to medical treatment. I do not feel obliged to make such proposals because all I have to presuppose for my considerations is that it is possible *in principle* to take the idea of an equal right to medical treatment as a meaningful guideline.

5
References

Breyer F, Kliemt H (1994) Lebensverlängernde medizinische Leistungen als Clubgüter? In: Homann K (ed) Wirtschaftsethische Perspektiven I. Berlin pp 131–58

Breyer F, Kliemt H (1995) Solidargemeinschaften der Organspender: Private oder öffentliche Organisation? In: Oberender P (ed) Transplantationsmedizin: Ökonomische, ethische, rechtliche und medizinische Aspekte. Baden-Baden, pp 135–160

Buchanan JM, Congleton RD (1998) Politics by Principle, Not Interest. Towards Nondicriminatory Democracy. Cambridge

De Jasay A (1991) Choice, Contract, Consent: A Restatement of Liberalism. London

Dworkin R (1978) Taking Rights Seriously. Cambridge MA

Kliemt H (1995) Life: What Is Worth Maintaining. In: Cardiovascular Risk Factors: An International Journal, Vol. 5, No. 4, August, pp 249–254

Kliemt H (1996) Rationierung im Gesundheitswesen als rechts-ethisches Problem. In: P. Oberender (ed) Rationalisierung und Rationierung im Gesundheitswesen, Gräfelfing, pp 23–31

Mackie JL (1978) Can There Be a Right-Based Moral Theory? In: Midwest Studies in Philosophy III, pp 350–359

Rawls J (1971) A Theory of Justice. Cambridge

Rationing – Basic Philosophical Principles and the Practice

Weyma Lübbe

"Rationing"* is a buzzword in a complex health policy debate. I use it here, but I will not spend time on the question as to how the term should be defined. The following paper, in any case, deals with the problem of a just allocation of medical resources which, for whatever reasons, are not available in sufficient quantity to cover all needs. The reason why a medical resource is not available in sufficient quantity is indeed often an allocational decision itself. The ethical status of such a decision should, or so it seems, be first discussed. I shall leave this out, for I am convinced that *any* reasonable decision on health budgets will, due to medical progress, lead to a budget that does not cover all needs – if not presently, then certainly in the near future. The question of what criteria should be used in political decisions on the limits of health budgets will therefore not be explicitly discussed here although some of the principles mentioned, being very general principles, do bear on questions of macroallocation.

Furthermore, I will concentrate, though not exclusively, on the allocation of life and death, including the risks of death. Thus, the important problem of prioritising various (more or less important, but not life-threatening) health needs is dropped as well. There is, in a certain sense, no more important health problem than death. But even if we strictly prioritised avoiding death, the problem of how to proceed when it comes to my death or your death, instead of my death or your health, would remain. If different answers are given to this question, their different basic commitments will influence the prioritising debate, too. Thus, I shall concentrate on the "Who shall survive?"-question because it is in this that certain basic ethical commitments which are relevant in all parts of the rationing debate can most clearly be discerned.

I will distinguish three well-known positions which dominate the philosophical debate on distributive justice and which are held to be relevant for the case of medical resources. They are utilitarianism, egalitarianism and libertarianism. I will of course not confine myself to just presenting them. Instead, it shall be demonstrated how they argue against each other. In doing so, I distinguish between arguments which, in my view, are cogent and those aspects of the debate which seem to me to require further clarification.

---

* Thanks for comments go to Michael Baurmann, Frank Dietrich, Christoph Fehige, Jacek Hołówka and Richard Raatzsch.

1
Utilitarianism

I define, for the present purpose, as "utilitarian"[1] a distribution procedure which aims for the maximisation of a certain value – e.g. the number of survivors, life years, "QALYs" – whereby that value is aggregated beyond the borders of persons. Indeed, utilitarians hold the claim that such procedures are not only efficient, i.e. maximising, but also just (after all, utilitarianism is a moral theory). The claim is founded on the argument that in the aggregating calculation anyone's gain of a unit of the reference value counts exactly the same. Thus, although the criticism that the allocation procedure lacks equity belongs to the standard objections to utilitarianism, this position indeed presents itself as a theory which holds to the value of equity.

Before discussing this claim, I shall present some practical examples. One maximising practice is the so-called *triage:* the sorting into urgency categories when one has to cope with sudden large numbers of injured persons. I quote a standard textbook on disaster medicine: The "aim of triage" is "to treat as many injured persons with a chance of survival as possible with the means available."[2] An example of a maximising approach from everyday medicine is the relevance of the prognosis (the likelihood of survival – sometimes also the quality of life – after treatment) when allocating transplants or places in intensive care units.

As these examples show, utilitarian criteria seem to be in use, and this quite openly and without causing any scandal. But this does not at all mean that the legitimacy of maximisation is generally undisputed. This is not even true for the reference value least attacked in the discussion – which is the number of survivors because in this case every life, independent of age and degree of incapacitation, counts the same. Since even when maximising the number of survivors, certain patients are systematically disadvantaged – in particular "expensive" patients, i.e. those whose survival requires a high input of resources. Even in the textbooks and manuals on disaster medicine (which is the most explicitly maximisation oriented medical practice), this group of patients does not appear as a separate sorting category[3] – which either means that disaster medicine is not really maximising the number of survivors, or else it means that the textbook authors prefer not to make this point explicit.

Thus, we have already arrived at the standard objection raised by the egalitarian counter position: The survival of any patient may well have been taken equally into

---

[1]   "Utilitarian" is, in fact, somewhat too specific with respect to the reference value while "consequentialist" is not specific enough. "Maximising" or "efficient" (in the economic sense of efficiency) at first sight fits better; but as we shall see, maximising procedures can be adopted on other than utilitarian grounds, too; so I use "utilitarian" because that is the label under which the problem of justice, being of interest in this section, has traditionally been debated.

[2]   Eberle (1980), p 30 (my translation).

[3]   For a detailed discussion, see Lübbe (2001), Veralltäglichung der Triage? Überlegungen zu Ausmaß und Grenzen der Opportunitätskostenorientierung in der Katastrophenmedizin und ihrer Übertragbarkeit auf die Alltagsmedizin.

account in the utilitarian calculation. But that in no way means equal chances of survival. On the contrary, it involves systematically unequal chances. How can one plausibly explain to the expensive patient, who now must die, that this is just? The standard utilitarian answer is: It is just because *more* persons can be saved in this way, and this is the best solution from an impartial point of view. Certainly it is not the best solution for the expensive patient. But the expensive patient, like everyone else, is expected to accept what is best from an impartial point of view.

Is this a cogent argument? As early as 1977, John Taurek, in a much cited essay,[4] called the argument into question in a way which, in my view, actually precludes supporting the "relevance of numbers" in the manner in which it has most often been supported up to this day. The supporters say that "precisely because each person's life is individually valuable, two lives are more valuable than one"[5] – and this they claim to be self-evident. Taurek shows why it is not.

Taurek's essay deals with the example of a life-saving drug which is only available in a limited quantity: Either one saves David, who needs the whole amount in order to survive, or one saves five other persons, each of whom can be helped with one fifth of the available quantity. I report only the central argument which Taurek presents for his thesis that the number of saved persons as such is not a morally relevant aspect. The argument is based upon a comparison between a rescue operation for people, on the one hand, and wooden figures, on the other hand. If someone is faced with the alternative of saving one precious wooden figure from one of the rooms of a burning house or of saving five equally precious figures from a different room, then he will choose the second room, because the five wooden figures are five times as precious to him as the one in the first room. In the case of a rescue operation involving people, it is, according to Taurek, generally a fundamentally different matter. The decision as to which persons are to be saved is not based upon their value for the rescuer but on the fact that the rescuer can sense the value that the persons themselves place upon their own lives: "It is the loss to the individual that matters to me, not the loss of the individual".[6] But if this is the case, then the loss wich occurred if five persons die is no greater than the loss if David dies since none of the five persons, *and no one else either*, suffers a greater loss than that which threatens David, namely the loss of his own life.

Thus, Taurek denies that from the pure fact that a condition will, numerically, involve more suffering we may conclude that this is the condition to be prevented from an objective point of view. Surely it is in no way, logically or otherwise, impossible to sum up "losses to" just as well as "losses of". But arguing with "losses to" makes explicit that the value of a life is a value *for* somebody in a sense in which the value of several lives is not. "More suffering *for whom?*" is the perpetual question which Taurek poses to the advocates of maximisation. "More suffering for all" is not the right answer since "all" includes David, too, who suffers less if the five others die. "More suffering for the other five" is unclear since the other five, collectively, are not a subjective entity and do not, therefore, suffer. "More suffer-

---

4   Taurek (1977), Do the Numbers Count?
5   Harris (1985), The Value of Life, p 21.
6   Taurek (1977), p 307.

ing for each of the five others" – that answer is wrong again, since each of the other five loses, like David, only his own life. To decide impartially, according to Taurek, thus means regarding the threat of any "loss to" as equally worthy of avoidance.[7] In other words, each threatened person should be offered an equal chance of survival. This would be respected, for example, by tossing a (fair) coin in order to decide whether to apply the whole supply of the drug to David or to use it to treat the other five.[8] Throwing a dice, instead, which might be the procedure springing to mind first, would give a chance of survival of one sixth to David and of five sixths to each of the other five since when David's number does not show up first he drops out because there will not be enough left to save him anyway.[9]

It appears to me that Taurek convincingly challenges the claim that he who sums up beyond the borders of persons is impartial.[10] In any case, it is much easier to part with this central element of utilitarianism if one sees that maximising does not *depend* on it: The next section will show that even if Taurek's understanding of impartiality is adopted it can still not be concluded that one must flip a coin – or that this, over and above that, is the solution for all similar cases, including, as the opponents promptly observed,[11] cases with billions of people standing on one of the two sides.

---

[7] Christoph Fehige claims that the higher value of the world in which David dies and the five others live follows from the Pareto-principle plus universalizability (private communication, referring to Fehige 1998, A Pareto Principle for Possible People, pp 527f). I do not think that "Pareto-superiority after role-swapping", as Fehige exemplifies it, can claim to incorporate impartiality in the way in which traditional applications of the principle of universalizability do. I hope to give a detailed critique on another occasion; the reader may form his own opinion in referring to the given quote and to Fehige's sources.

[8] Taurek (1977), p 306.

[9] Jacek Hołówka, referring to Szaniawski (1979), On Formal Aspects of Distributive Justice, has argued that assigning a number to each of the six persons, throwing a dice and letting the winner take what he needs is impartial while also doing justice to intuitions concerning efficiency: "I believe that people should be given equal chances, and I could even swallow the phrase 'numbers do not count', but I would give it a different twist. Numbers do not count in the sense that when people associate and form a group they still count each as one, and not as a group, i.e. they should be separately represented on the dice" (private communication). But "equal chances", in that case, are not "equal chances to survive" (or "equal chances of satisfaction", see Szaniawski, pp 137ff) *nor* are they "equal chances of choice" (see Szaniawski, pp 141ff). They are merely equal chances to have the *first* choice. These two differ because David, unlike the others, does not have a chance to make his choice (i.e. to take what is a good for him, see Szaniawski, p 136) as the winner of a second, third etc. throwing of the dice. Szaniawksi, in his paper, does not discuss a case in which not having the first choice definitely means getting no good at all for some of the participants while others have a chance of making their choices later. Of course one can stick to the position that, in the David-case, providing equal chances of getting the *first* choice is "just enough", i.e. in view of a wish to do justice (if one may say so) to efficiency intuitions, too. For another line of argument to that effect which does not violate the principle of equality of chances (to survive), see section 2.

[10] See, for further discussion, Parfit (1978), Innumerate Ethics, Rakowski (1991), Equal Justice, ch. 12, Kamm (1993), Morality, Mortality, ch. 5, 6, Scanlon (1998), What We Owe to Each Other, pp 230–241.

[11] For instance, Sanders (1988), Why the Numbers Should Sometimes Count, pp 3f.

2
Egalitarianism

The standard egalitarian objection to utilitarianism (in the context of rationing at least) is not that equal needs are not met equally. In most cases it is not possible to allocate scarce medical resources in such a way that needs are met equally, i.e. – since there is a scarcity – partially, namely equally partially for all. Many medical goods, for example rescue helicopters, are not divisible. Others are divisible, e.g. the drug in the Taurek example, but if you administer it in equal relation to each patient's needs, all of them will die. Taurek's egalitarian solution, therefore, does not aim at equal fulfilment of needs but at affording the same *chances* of need fulfilment.

Accordingly, egalitarians normally accept the transition from equality of results to equality of chances. Thus they, too, (not only the utilitarians) normatively expect the patients to accept unequal fulfilment of needs. Here, too, some patients die while others survive. Why should all patients consider this to be just? One possible answer is: The agreement to inequality of result can be based upon an ex ante consent – in Taurek's case, for example, on an agreement to toss the coin.[12] Also, the acceptance of this procedure – or so it appears – must not be prescribed normatively. It will occur of its own since, unlike the actual result of the coin tossing, the adoption of the procedure is in everyone's own interest. To be more precise (and we shall come back to this reservation presently): the adoption of the procedure is in everyone's own interest as long as it is in everyone's interest that the scarce good is allocated in a consented way – and not, say, by stealing or fighting.

Thus, in classical philosophical terms, the egalitarian position may be based on contract theory. That means it also entails all the problems of this approach. The most fundamental of these was addressed by Hobbes. He passed on to us the question of whether contracts are binding (i.e. whether breach of contract is unjust), if adherence to the contract runs contrary to the end on which the consent to the contract was based. According to Hobbes, it can never be presupposed that someone has bound himself to a contract which entails renouncing his self-preservation.[13] But that is exactly what is implied if one claims that the loser should accept the outcome when drawing lots in cases of life and death. Certainly the loser cannot object that this claim is unjust. But he can withdraw from participation in the

---

[12] See the contract theoretical considerations Taurek (using another example) adds to his argument against the relevance of numbers (1977, pp 310 ff).

[13] See for instance Hobbes (1651), Leviathan, p 66, pp 69 f. Literally, the text reads that a "covenant not to defend my selfe from force, by force, is alwayes voyd" (p 70). It might be questioned whether, according to Hobbes, this idea extends to cases where self-preservation does not require defence, but attack (like in a fight for a resource which is in the hands of someone else). But the reasons which Hobbes gives for the impossibility of a covenant not to defend oneself seem to apply to both cases: "For ... no man can ... lay down his Right to save himself from Death ... the avoyding whereof is the onely End of laying down any Right ..." and "For man by nature chooseth the lesser evill" (p 70).

discourse on justice. Talk of "justice" and "injustice" is made by and for those who are interested in such talk. For this reason Hobbes refrains from declaring unjust those who, in the face of death, no longer go along with an agreement.[14]

It seems to me that Hobbes' point is, within his premises, consistent and that it has some practical relevance. The truth of the old saying "necessitas non habet legem" has found its expression in law as well – in the German penal code, for instance, in § 35, concerning pardonable behaviour in cases of emergency. The first sentence of the first section reads: "Anyone who in the event of immediate and otherwise unavoidable danger for life, limb or freedom commits an act against the law in order to avert danger from himself, from a relative or from another person close to him acts without blame". I have occasionally busied myself with the question of how textbooks and commentaries on this subject tone down the explosive content of this sentence – for instance in a case where someone deprived of receiving an expensive medical drug by a rationing programme procures it by force. None of the authors referred to were as radical as Hobbes.[15]

Thus, we may accept that also in the case of an egalitarian rationing programme the consent of the loser to the outcome can not be taken for granted – and, what is more, it can not even be unambiguously demonstrated that he who does not consent is unjust. If one does not opt out of the discourse on justice, for whatever reasons, the possibility remains to fight for survival within it, i.e. with arguments. The egalitarian theory, as we have seen, holds that unequal chances in meeting health needs are unjust. How is it then that persons with an unpromising prognosis (or their relatives) do not protest when the place in the intensive care unit is given to a fellow patient with a better prognosis? The utilitarian answer – it is better if one tries to save the most saveable – is, as we saw, not wholly convincing. (*For whom* is it better if one tries to save the most saveable? For the one with the better prognosis.) Here is another explanation: Taking account of the prognosis, and many other efficiency-oriented allocation procedures, does not conflict as such with the principle of equality of chances. That depends rather on the point of time chosen to obtain the ex ante consent.

The following example will promptly clarify what is meant. Let us consider two heart attack patients. A, the one with the bad prognosis, and B, the one with the better prognosis, may be asked which allocation procedure with regard to places in intensive care units they would accept. Yet, it can make a difference whether they are asked *before* or *after* their heart attacks. Assume that A and B, before their heart attacks, have no recognizably different chances of a bad prognosis. In this epistemic situation, there would be no violation of the principle of equality of chances

---

[14] In Hobbesian terms, it remains unclear whether an agreement to draw lots in cases of life and death could have been made at all. There is clearly, ex ante, an incentive to make it when the stakes for survival are better than in a fight for the resource (so there is "some Good to himselfe" to be achieved by each contracting party as Hobbes requires (1651, p 66)). But, again ex ante, it can not be believed that the loser will keep the agreement – so it must be considered to be void from the start.

[15] See, for much relevant material, Bernsmann (1989), "Entschuldigung" durch Notstand, who himself advocates a more extensive reading of the excuse conditions than most authors; for discussion of health resource examples see p 20, pp 50–52 and especially pp 359–367.

if a decision were made to give preference to the (future) patient with the better prognosis. A common argument adds that A and B, if they were reasonable, would actually decide that way because this is the allocation procedure which, as far as they can see, maximises their personal chances of survival. Our practical example, the triage of disaster medicine, also submits to this logic: One cannot not know beforehand whether, in the event of a disaster, one will belong to the slightly or to the severely injured persons. Thus, one maximises one's chances of survival if one agrees to an allocation procedure which gives priority to the severely wounded.

Evidently, the concept of ex ante consent can lead to maximising allocation procedures without having to rely on a utilitarian way of reasoning (i.e. on the contention that values should be summed up beyond the borders of persons).[16] I think that this explains why maximising procedures meet with more acceptance in practice than utilitarianism does in theory. We must remember, however, the aforementioned problem: Whether maximising procedures are in accordance with the principle of equality of chances depends on the point of time at which ex ante consent is obtained. Which point of time, then, is the point to choose?

The most obvious answer seems to be this: The real point of time is the time to choose. One has to keep to the epistemic situation that actually exists at the time when the decision regarding the allocation procedure has to be made. Which point of time is that, say, in the case of the heart attack example? Of course, the decision concerning the allocation of places in intensive care units is not made according to the acute needs of A and B but according to the interests of all persons possibly concerned by the procedure. But the time for the decision can actually happen to coincide with the moment at which A and B are delivered to hospital. In other words, at any possible time when such a decision is made, there will be someone who now has an unfavourable prognosis, or, more generally speaking, who knows presently that he belongs to those who will lose when a maximising procedure is adopted. Can we normatively expect such patients to imagine themselves at some earlier point in time when they were still healthy – arguing that they now have to admit that they would have wished to have a maximising procedure and would have considered it to be just if they had been asked at that earlier point in time?

I believe that an exhaustive discussion of this question is important for the future of rationing but that it is also very difficult. Partly for reasons of space and partly because of uncertainties remaining to me, I confine myself here to a number of observations.

1. The answer that one simply *was* not asked earlier does not strike me as convincing. It is plausible when – as in Hobbes's contract – it is a matter of the

---

[16] The possibility of a "utilitarianism from behind the veil of ignorance" is of course well known in the recent debate on distributive justice – see Roemer (1996), commenting on Harsanyi (1977) and others. Differences occur with respect to the question whether, based upon ex ante-consent, maximising is still "utilitarian" (I do not mind the word as long as it is clear that there is no arguing with values summed up beyond the borders of persons). More important differences occur 1. with respect to the question whether consent is (always) to be given under an *artificial*, i.e. normatively prescribed veil of ignorance concerning one's own position, and 2. with respect to the question whether rational individuals will (always) maximise their expected utilities. See further remarks below.

transition from the natural state to the social state. But that is not our point of departure today when discussing rationing. It really cannot be said that in the question of rationing nothing is valid in our societies until everyone has agreed to it. The Constitutional Law, for instance, including the competences in decision-making stipulated therein, is already there. In other words, anyone who takes up the position that procedures of rationing depend on his actual consent is not different from Hobbes's individual who does not go along with an earlier agreement when times get rough. Such an individual, as mentioned before, should not be described as unjust. But one does not have to allow oneself to be described as unjust either when one nevertheless lets him die.[17]

2. Considerably stronger is the position of the patient who can say that at no earlier time was he ever in a position in which he was not disadvantaged by the maximising procedure. This holds true for persons born ill – and it explains (and substantiates, too) why this group, including many handicapped persons, is fundamentally opposed to proposals to give second priority to expensive patients, to patients with a lower expected quality of life, and so on.

3. The concept of risk aversion – well-known from the debate about Rawls – cannot support turning away from efficiency when it is a matter of life and death. The concept expounds that reasonable people do not pay heed to maximising their expected outcomes when granting ex ante consent, but that instead they are concerned with maximising the worst possible condition in which they might end up. But if the worst possible condition to be allocated is death anyway, there is nothing to be maximised – except, of course, the chance that one will not be hit by it. On the other hand, risk aversion is indeed relevant insofar as rationing is not about life or death but about better or worse degrees of health.[18] Then it provides an argument for proposals which prioritise giving resources to those whose state of health is nearest to death (but something, evidently, will have to be added on how much a difference the allocation of the resource makes for the health state in question).

4. Classical decision theory holds that the rational individual seeks to maximise her expected outcome – which means that when uncertain about her future she banks on an efficient allocation of resources. This explication of rationality has been called into question in several respects. Empirical psychological studies and, by the way, also the decision practice in the health system, in particular in the field of prevention, show that we often do not stick to that concept of rationality. Whether that speaks against us or against the concept is a subject of dispute. The answer, in my opinion, must also depend on whether individuals who are otherwise regarded as reasonable may be convinced into taking the "rational" option by a thorough explanation of the fact that they are reducing their expected outcomes. In so far as they cannot be convinced, decision theory is faced with the task of explaining the discrepancy. In this field, as far as I can

---

[17] When Hobbes says that the criminal who tries to elope when condemned to death is not unjust even when he earlier consented to the law by which he was condemned, he obviously does not want to say that the sovereign is unjust unless he lets him elope; see Hobbes 1651, p 70.

[18] The question gets more complicated again if the number of expected life years is added as a relevant value.

see, very much is still quite unclear, and as long as this is the case, we should not generally assume that any rational being will give her ex ante consent to maximising allocation procedures.

In order to illustrate this point, I shall recount two classical examples. The first one I cite from Jonathan Glover.[19] It refers to a decision problem which apparently really occurred among bomber pilots on missions during the second world war: "At a certain place, a pilot's chances of surviving his thirty bombing missions were only one in four. It was calculated that one-way missions, by reducing the fuel load, could increase the load of bombs, so that only half the pilots need fly. Selection would be by lot, with half the pilots escaping altogether and half going to certain death. On this system, fatalities would be halved, but it was not adopted." The second example is fictitious – but the inventor, from his position, has no clue why. I refer to John Harris's "survival lottery":[20] We could join a club in which, whenever two or more of us needed a transplant, one member could be selected by drawing lots to serve as donor. So far no such club exists – although it would improve the survival chances of the members. This is certainly not due to technical problems alone nor is it merely a result of the paternalistic standpoint of the legislator either.

The relevant points in these two examples are discussed in different contexts under the headings "individual versus statistical life"[21] and "killing versus letting die"[22] respectively, and they are, in my opinion, highly relevant for the

---

[19] Glover (1977), Causing Death and Saving Lives, p 212.

[20] Harris (1994), The Survival Lottery (first 1975).

[21] See Linnerooth (1982), Murdering Statistical Lives …?, Krämer (1988), Der statistische Wert eines Menschenlebens; see also the early remarks in Glover (1977), pp 210–213, and Menzel (1983), Medical Costs, Moral Choices, pp 151–183, especially pp 159–163. One of the many problems of this distinction is that there is no clear dividing line between the two concepts, rather a continuous scale: people may be more or less individualised, depending on the size of the statistical group concerned by a macroallocative decision. Is, for instance, a decision of the Oregon kind (some 30 transplant patients being denied help in favour of the inclusion of several thousand people in the basic health care) a decision on "statistical lives"? The transplant patients must have thought that they were being allowed to die quite individually.

[22] It might be thought that the killing/letting die-debate is not important for the rationing problem because rationing is only about letting die anyway – and not about killing. But there are at least two reasons why it is relevant: firstly, rationing is not only about letting die but sometimes about withdrawing aid as well – and whether or under what circumstances that amounts to killing is not at all a simple question; see, for the general debate, McMahan (1994), Killing, Letting Die and Withdrawing Aid; for some hints to examples relevant for the rationing practice see Lübbe (2001); secondly, and more fundamentally: except from cases of withdrawing aid, rationing is, up to now, indeed not about killing. But if we want – against consequentialism – to justify why it should not be, either, then we have to discuss the moral relevance of the distinction. Why, for instance, do we (in case we still do) hold the position that a person may live on with her healthy organs when she does so "over their dead bodies" (Harris 1994, p 262) – the bodies of those four or five persons one could have saved by dividing that resource? For most participants in the rationing debate, the right to one's own body is too self-evident to need justification. But all I want to say, for now, is that this talk of rights – and a fortiori the libertarian position on rationing to be discussed in the next section – depends on the moral relevance of the distinction between killing and letting die; and this relevance is heavily attacked in theory. It may also be added that there are debates in medical

subject of rationing. More, or so it seems to me, should be said about both points in the theoretical and in the applied debate.

3
Libertarianism

Libertarianism does not share the egalitarian idea that justice has to do with equality – with equal chances just as little as with equal results. Libertarians, instead, promote "justice in transfer" – as it was called by Robert Nozick.[23] His starting point is what indeed we see to be true in practice: By far the majority of goods already belong to someone. Therefore, there is no allocation problem. "Justice in transfer" means that certain rules concerning the transfer of property positions are adhered to. Thus, making gifts, bequeathing, inheriting, buying and selling – including buying of insurance policies – are legitimate but not theft. This is also widely confirmed by looking at what takes place in practice – not, however, in regard to one's own organs.

There are other respects in which the libertarian position does not coincide with what happens in practice: Compulsory levies are regarded as unwarranted incursions upon the rights of the citizen. This holds also for levies that are used to help persons who have not taken precautions for their own health or (and this amounts to the same thing) who were unable to take precautions. Thus, a desolate situation of need as such in no way justifies a redistribution of goods. However, there is justification if the situation of need was preceded by having suffered damage – here one has a claim against the person who caused the damage. The violation of contracts – among these insurance contracts – is just one special case of damage. The difference between damaging and merely not helping corresponds to the traditional distinction between *iustitia* and *caritas*: *iustitia*, justice, demands that one does not take away what belongs to another (or that one gives it back); it does not demand that one rectifies the results of fate.

Such are the basic commitments of this position. Although it seems to have nothing in common with the egalitarian position, the most relevant difference can be localised at one point: Libertarianism recognises pre-contractual entitlements. To possess rights is not in all cases held to be the result of mutual consent. In particular (the classical reference for this is Locke)[24], every person has a natural and exclusive right to her own body. Non-libertarian theoreticians regard this as unjust since it means being bound, without compensation, to a resource, the condition of which varies by nature. It seems all the more unjust because these natural differences, via the libertarian theory of acquiring property (which is based on working), involve differences in the ability to raise one's state of health with the help of one's property.

---

practice in which the self-evident nature of the right to one's own body is at least partly called into question (viz. the debate about medical research without the consent of the patient and without medical use to him).

23 Nozick (1974), Anarchy, State, and Utopia, p 150.
24 Locke (1993) Two Treatises of Government, § 27, p 128.

The discussion shows that, with regard to the following three categories of health differences, agreement between libertarians and egalitarians is, in principle, not difficult to achieve: Firstly, regarding those differences which are determined by unequal *use* of opportunities which were equal. In the following, I call this category of health differences "self-inflicted". These differences, under aspects of justice, do not warrant a claim to compensation (I shall come to what happens in practice presently). Secondly, those differences which are outcomes of unequal *luck* insofar as the risk has been, ex ante, equal and consented. This includes all examples for which ex ante consent, as discussed earlier, can be presupposed – such as the case in which A, after a heart attack, finds himself to be the patient with the bad prognosis. I put these cases under the heading "consented chance". These, too, do not warrant a claim to compensation. Thirdly, and at first sight the least disputed, those health inequalities that result from damage inflicted by others – in this case a claim to compensation exists against these others.

The only disputed category remaining, so it would seem, are those differences determined by non-consented chance – in particular, indeed, the inborn differences. The classical antagonists in the relevant discussion are Rawls[25] and Nozick. Nozick holds that a problem of just allocation only exists with respect to the cooperative gain (he is referring to the surplus which is achieved by the division of labour), not with regard to the input which everyone brings into the cooperation – including one's own natural talents.[26] However, the concept of cooperative gain can not be limited to the surplus derived from the division of labour. It covers, in addition, that one may *keep* what one has been given by nature. In other words, it is already a cooperative gain if the less well-endowed accept the alleged natural rights. Their acceptance will, possibly, not be given for nothing. So, at this point, too, the threat of not cooperating, which includes the threat of being killed in the fight for resources, is lurking behind the talk of "rights". Of course, if that threat came from those born ill or with handicaps alone, it would not have made much effect. But it never came from that side alone.

That is at least in part due to difficulties of clearly distinguishing the afore-mentioned categories of ascribing responsibility for health inequalities in practice. The judgement that a certain health problem is self-inflicted would involve immensely complex problems of imputation if we really wanted to do away with all differences in abilities or opportunities which have been laid by non-consented chance. It is no easier, at second sight, to make sound judgements on whether a health problem is "inflicted by others". There are countless health differences which are due to differences in the environment caused by others, but the law of damages does not count them as inflicted harm – while the harm is evidently not natural, nor is it self-inflicted. Be that as it may – in practice, the tackling of these knotty problems of ascribing responsibility will be put off as long as possible. Rationing programmes demanding that the aforesaid categories be consistently considered and adhered to are, therefore, currently still having a hard time in practice – as well as in theory.

---

[25] Rawls (1971), A Theory of Justice.
[26] See Nozick (1974), especially pp 183 ff.

So, in which direction should rationing go? Ideally, it seems this way: 1. Further attempt must be made to clarify the remaining problems involved in the discourse of justice – since there are, as I believe, aspects of the debate which *can* profit from further analysis. 2. A rationing programme acceptable according to the state of the art in the current debate must be worked out and be decided on. Since the state of the art in the debate, at present and, in my opinion, in the future as well, does not, even under the most ideal conditions (i.e. with everybody honestly striving for justice), filter out one procedure as the only acceptable rationing procedure, there must be political decision-making involved, i.e. the procedure can not be expected to rest on nothing more than good arguments for exactly that procedure. 3. One must hope that there is acceptance to the unavoidable schematisation involved in the implementation of any programme as well. 4. One should stick to what has been decided when the media present a delightful little six-year-old who happens to need the very resource that one has refused to make generally available.

If the question is instead: Where *will* rationing go?, then there are other possibilities. The most likely one – and the one that will certainly materialise partly in addition to any future explicit rationing programme – has been described by Calabresi and Bobbit under the heading "The Customary or Evolutionary Approach":[27] The pressure towards rationing discharges itself in the dark corners of inattentiveness and it hits those incapable or unwilling to protest and to argue. This may be accompanied by what social scientists (possibly overrating the intentionality of the process) call "value management"[28]: The conflict of values, so they say, is concealed behind all kinds of vague terminology and the ample use of quasi-objective, medical-sounding terminology. Then the patients, halfway pacified, will lie back and leave the experts to make the decisions. This, if not just, is perhaps merciful: It is, after all, easier to die from medical causes then for reasons of justice.

4
References

Calabresi G, Bobbitt P (1978) Tragic Choices. The Conflicts Society Confronts in the Allocation of Tragically Scarce Resources. W. W. Norton & Co, New York/London

Bernsmann K (1989) "Entschuldigung" durch Notstand. Carl Heymanns, Köln

Eberle H (1980) Triage. In: Lanz R, Rossetti M (eds) Katastrophenmedizin. Fedinand Enke, Stuttgart, pp 29–33

Fehige (1998), Christoph, A Pareto Principle for Possible People. In: Fehige C, Wessels U (eds) Preferences. Walter de Gruyter, Berlin/New York, pp 508–543

Feuerstein G (1995) Das Transplantationssystem. Dynamik, Konflikte und ethisch-moralische Grenzgänge. Juventa, Weinheim/München

Feuerstein G, Kollek R (1999) Flexibilisierung der Moral. Zum Verhältnis von biotechnischen Innovationen und ethischen Normen. In: Claudia Honegger et al. (eds), Grenzenlose Gesellschaft?, vol. 2. Leske & Budrich, Opladen, pp 559–574

---

[27] Calabresi, Bobbitt (1978), Tragic Choices, p 44–49.

[28] Feuerstein, Kollek (1999), Flexibilisierung der Moral, p 573; see, for the case of organ allocation, Schmidt, Hartmann (1997), Lokale Gerechtigkeit in Deutschland, ch. 4, and Feuerstein (1995), Das Transplantationssystem, especially ch. VI.2.

Glover J (1977) Causing Death and Saving Lives, Penguin, London

Harris J (1985) The Value of Life. An Introduction to Medical Ethics. Routledge & Kegan Paul, London

Harris J (1994) The Survival Lottery. In: Steinbock B, Norcross A (eds) Killing and Letting Die, 2nd ed. Fordham, New York, pp 257–265

Harsanyi JC (1977) Rational Behavior and Bargaining Equilibrium in Games and Social Situations. Cambridge UP, Cambridge

Hobbes T (1651) Leviathan or The Matter, Forme and Power of a Commonwealth Ecclesiasticall and Civil. London (repr. Oxford: Clarendon 1929)

Kamm, FM (1993) Morality, Mortality. Vol. I: Death and Whom to Save from It. Oxford UP, New York/Oxford

Krämer W (1988) Der statistische Wert eines Menschenlebens. In: Medizin Mensch Gesellschaft 13, pp 34–41

Linnerooth J (1982) Murdering Statistical Lives …? In: Michael W. Jones-Lee (ed) The Value of Life and Safety. North-Holland Publishing Company, Amsterdam, pp 229–261

Locke J (1993) Two Treatises of Government. Everyman, London/Vermont

Lübbe W (2001) Veralltäglichung der Triage? Überlegungen zu Ausmaß und Grenzen der Opportunitätskostenorientierung in der Katastrophenmedizin und ihrer Übertragbarkeit auf die Alltagsmedizin. In: Ethik in der Medizin (forthcoming)

McMahan J (1994) Killing, Letting Die, and Withdrwaing Aid. In: Steinbock B, Norcross A (eds) Killing and Letting Die, 2nd ed. Fordham, New York, pp 383–420

Menzel PT (1983) Medical Costs, Moral Choices. Yale UP, New Haven/London

Nozick R (1974) Anarchy, State, and Utopia. Blackwell, Oxford/Cambridge

Parfit D (1978) Innumerate Ethics. In: Philosophy and Public Affairs 7, pp 285–301

Rakowski E (1991) Equal Justice. Clarendon, Oxford

Rawls J (1971) A Theory of Justice. Clarendon, Oxford

Roemer JE (1996) Theories of Distributive Justice. Harvard UP, Cambridge, Mass.

Sanders JT (1988) Why the Numbers Should Sometimes Count. In: Philosophy and Public Affairs 17, pp 3–14

Scanlon TM (1998) What We Owe to Each Other. Belknap, Cambridge Mass./London

Schmidt VH, Hartmann BK (1997) Lokale Gerechtigkeit in Deutschland. Studien zur Verteilung von Bildungs-, Arbeits- und Gesundheitsgütern. Westdeutscher Verlag, Opladen

Szaniawski K (1979) On Formal Aspects of Distributive Justice. In: Saarinen E, Hilpinen R, Provence Hintikka MB (eds) Essays in Honour of Jaako Hintikka. D. Reidel, Dordrecht, pp 135–146 (original polish version in 1966)

Taurek JM (1977) Should the Numbers Count? In: Philosophy and Public Affairs 6, pp 293–316

IV   The Future of Rationing

Complementarity of Private and Public Insurance

Jürgen Fritze

The request for health care services is in principle unlimited because life usually ends with a kind of death to which illness precedes. Request is additionally unlimited because in the context of the generally changing appraisal the general and scientific conceptions change of what might be an illness in need of treatment as opposed to complaints and changes of the state of health to be tolerated. Moreover, request is unlimited because medical progress (driven by medical need and also scientific curiosity) opens ever new possibilities of treatment. It is finally unlimited because owing to general welfare and medical progress the prevalences of chronic diseases, i.e. diseases continuously in need of treatment, increase. It is plausible that the unlimited request cannot be satisfied in health care systems where ressources are supplied on the basis of the principle of solidarity, i.e. where the individual access to health services is unlimited while the individual financial contribution is limited by the individual capability. This applies irrespective of whether the solidary health care system is financed by taxes or sick fund contributions.

Thus, rationing of health care services is inevitable in solidary health care systems although this is still officially not admitted or ignored e.g. in Germany. Covert rationing has been taking place for long as exemplified by the relation between the ressources provided by the budgets (fig. 1) and the actual expenses (fig. 2) for outpatient drug treatment on the one hand and the number of SHI-authorized physicians on the other in German counties. Although being somewhat strange this relationship represents the only detectable logic to explain the variability of the budgets and expenses, respectively, between German counties, and the relationship is plausible: The higher the number of prescribers the higher the total budget within each county; the more the budget thus grows the more increases the (political) pressure to dampen this growth; this finally results in considerably lower budgets per citizen although this seems medically bizarre.

The necessity of rationing is obviously although only implicitly accepted by the public in that the majoritiy of the people as represented by the majority in parliament supports the actual restriction of the contributions to statutory sick funds. Indeed, the idea to contribute an ever increasing share of income to the sick funds is no real option because in terms of opportunity costs every citizen has additional and possibly conflicting preferences although health is ranking highest as evidenced by several polls. Moreover, contributions are payed by the majority of healthy people while about 80 per cent of ressources are consumed by only 20 per cent of the population. Thus, there is also a conflict of interests between healthy and sick people. Nevertheless, the question is unresolved and still not really publicly disputed which share of income provided for solidary health care might be medically and economically adequate and individually acceptable in terms of the willingness to pay.

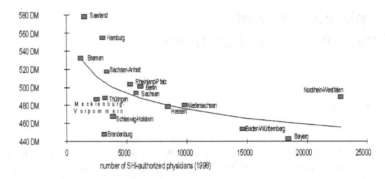

Fig. 1. Budgets for outpatient drug treatment and dressings (1999) per citizen insured by the statutory health insurance in relation to the number of SHI-authorized physicians (1998) in German states

Admittedly, however, this question cannot be answered in isolation because the range of the share provided for health care will depend on international competitiveness in the globalized economy.

While the supply of resources under the principle of solidarity is based on current-income financing with vertical redistribution between age groups and horizontal redistribution between groups of income, private insurance is based on individualized charges principally equivalent to the financial risks to be covered. Thus, in principle, the lifetime sum of fees will equal the sum of health care expenses in private health insurance irrespective of the individual economic capacity although there is some horizontal and vertical redistribution. There is no doubt that the principle of solidarity in the interest of those citizens in need of protection is ethically indispensable so that the option of private health insurances has to be restricted to the higher income groups.

If we, then, for ethical reasons adhere to the principle of solidarity, limitations of services, i.e. rationing, have to also be ethically justified. The basic, decisive ethical requirement is that the rules governing the limitations, i.e. rationing, are transparent and that the criteria for which services are to be excluded from reimbursement are not arbitrary. The only way to avoid arbitraryness is to base the exclusion criteria on sound scientific evidence. The evidence to be considered includes among others epidemiological data on morbidity and mortality; efficacy, effectiveness and efficiency (costs) of treatment options; acceptability and utilization of treatment options; and quality of life. The scientific input, however, is only a necessary but not sufficient requirement because medical science can only provide some order of services ranking from indispensable for survival to optimal for well-being. Medical science can, however, not provide the cut-off point. Therefore, in addition, a public consensus has to be developed where to set the cut-off. This public dispute is only going to start. Services excluded by public consense from reimbursement by statutory sick funds, then, might be of interest for coverage by some complementary private health insurance.

In principle, private health insurance might cover the whole spectrum of health risks and thus be substitutive to other insurances or it might be complementary in

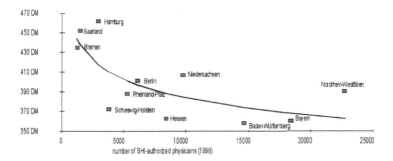

Fig. 2. Expenses for outpatient drug treatment and dressings (1998) per citizen insured by the statutory health insurance in relation to the number of SHI-authorized physicians (1998) in German states

that it covers risks not covered by other, e.g. statutory insurances. The access to a fully substitutive private health insurance is restricted by law in that only those whose income by dependent occupation exceeds a certain amount fixed by government have free choice between private and statutory insurance. At present, 6,2 Mill. of the population have chosen statutory insurance although they fulfill the criteria for free choice, most probably because the statutory insurance grants coverage for all family members without additional charges (so-called family insurance).

There are several possibilities for the option of complementarity all of which are already utilized today:

i)   in case of hospital treatment, private insurance might cover the claim for services other patients receive only by chance or by medical neccessity, i.e. some kind of comfort or specific quality like single room accomodation or treatment by the head of the medical department (who is expected to possess most expertise);

ii) it might cover in a more global manner costs in case another insurance grants coverage only for a certain limited amount or percentage of total costs;

iii) it might cover specific risks deliberately excluded from coverage by other, e.g. statutory insurances.

Thus, the question of complementarity of private health insurances to statutory health insurances (sick funds) is not new but might get additional drive in case that overt rationing would be introduced in the public sector. The option mentioned last is the one addressed in case of overt rationing, and – while secret rationing is a common phenomenon – there are also examples for private coverage of risks excluded from statutory insurances, i.e. overt rationing.

Complementarity of the private and public sector is quite common today in Germany and might even be thought to represent more the rule than the exception: At present, about 14,8 Mill. German citizens, i.e. 18 per cent of the population have signed one or the other mode of private health insurance. In less than half of them, i.e. 7,206 Mill. or 8,8 per cent, the private health insurance is substitutive to statutory insurance in that it covers the complete spectrum of health problems.

In about half of the latter group private health insurance covers some part of health expenses in that it is complementary in terms of the second option: Public servants are granted free of charge a limited sickness support the degree of which varies depending on various, individual conditions. Public servants supplement this limited coverage accordingly by a complementary private health insurance (although they are not obliged to do), thus optionally completing their coverage to 100 per cent of total costs. Almost 88 per cent (6,3 Mill.) of those with a full coverage insurance (including public servants) have additionally chosen tariffs covering one or the other additional service for in-patient treatment (first option). Additionally, about 4,4 Mill. people insured in the sick funds make use of this option.

There are also examples for the third option: 4,5 Mill. people have covered one or the other risk not included in statutory health insurance. The most prominent and recent example is the coverage for artificial teeth in children and adolescents. This rationing has been reversed by the government meanwhile.

Obviously, principally every health risk can be insured in the private sector. But as part of a free market private insurance companies cannot be forced to offer insurances for every risk. The fundamental question and limiting factor is whether coverage can be offered at charges attractive to the population and affordable to the insurer. The basis for calculating charges is that the sum of charges payed by the clients during their lifetime equals the costs of the specific treatment insured multiplied by the probability with which the specific risk is expected to occur. The less clearcut the idea of the size of this probability is, i.e. the less we know about this risk from e.g. epidemiology, the higher the charges will be. The attractiveness of such tariffs will certainly decrease with increasing charges. This may well lead to the selection of a high risk population covered by this tariff. The resultingly decreasing "dilution" of risks will necessarily require a further increase of the charges needed. Thus, it is quite reasonable to assume that there will be health risks where the charges for coverage are unaffordable to the population. At the end, this might mean that no insurance for this specific risk will be offered.

Other major obstacles to a complementary private insurance of specific risks may result from further uncertainties for the insurers concerning their capabilities to control usage. Whenever a complementary insurance is designed as an add-on to a more basic insurance, utilization tends to depend on and to be sanctioned by the confirmation of coverage by the respective basic insurance company, e.g. the statutory sick fund. Thus, as prominent and actual examples, there is hardly a real chance to refuse coverage of single room accommodation or personal treatment by the head of department if the basic insurance (e.g. in public servants) has granted coverage and thus acknowledged the medical necessity of the intervention. Similar constellations are quite conceivable where medical risks are covered complementarily.

This may be illustrated by the following – admittedly extreme – example which is based on the model of rationing established in the United Kingdom: If a complementary insurance promises coverage of dialysis in renal insufficiency at the age of over 65 years a patient suffering a myocardial infarction with treatment resistent intermittent ventricular fibrillation leading to the implantation of a defibrillator device and resuscitation which due to delay leaves the patient with an apallic syndrome and persistent renal insufficiency may well be faced with the costs of dialysis for another 20 years. If the defibrillator (covered by the basic insurance) had not been implanted which is suggested to be disputable in this constellation the patient whould have died.

Moreover, there are further hurdles related to the term medical necessity. If not otherwise agreed upon in the policy, private health insurance owes reimbursement for all medically necessary treatment. Although poorly defined the term of medical necessity as an approximation is meant as to demarcate optimal and desirable services. It implicates all measures necessary to identify and cure an illness, to prevent its progression or to alleviate complaints. Thus, treatment is medically necessary if an illness is present, if the diagnostic measures are scientifically adequate to clarify its origin and to confirm the diagnosis, if the therapeutic measures deduced from diagnostic findings are suitable to predictably cure the illness or at least improve the condition or prevent its progression or alleviate symptoms and complaints. Suitability in this context is meant as efficacy, tolerability and safety established according to scientific standards.

Nevertheless, this tentative definition leaves open the connotations of what might be an illness. These connotations are subject to change in that inceasingly more or less trivial discomforts or impairments previously allocated to the realm of private life are increasingly assumed to represent a true illness. Treatment options concerned comprise e.g. the field of so-called life-style drugs and accupuncture. Health care services excluded from reimbursement by statutory sick funds in accordance with the principles of scientific soundness and public consense outlined above will most probably and preferencially address services related to such fields. It is to be expected that consumers will utilize such services more or less unconscionably if these are covered by an insurance. The possibilities of the insurer to manage this utilization are – by definition – rather limited in these fields. This, again, means hardly manageable economic risks to the insurance.

In conclusion, in case of the implementation of overt rationing there is certainly an option for private health insurers to complementarily cover health risks left uncovered by statutory health insurances. Such options will, however, be limited by economic hurdles, i.e. if the charges needed to grant coverage are unattractive or even unaffordable to people.

Rationing of Health Care and the Complementarity of Private and Public Insurance

Achim Wambach

Rising expenditures in the health care sector has put the public health insurance system under pressure to reduce costs and thus to ration health care. Consequently the question arises if and how private health insurance might cover services which the public system will no longer provide. In the following, I will discuss this interplay between private and public health insurance in the context of rationing of health care. In particular, three aspects will be considered:

First, I will ask the question whether private insurers should not rather substitute public insurance – what is the reason for governmental intervention? It is my opinion that we first have to understand why we would like to have public health insurance, before we can discuss what limits the system should have. Based on this analysis I will then in a second step outline what economic theory has to say about rules for rationing. In a third step, I will speculate how such a (theoretically devised) system might evolve.

Let me start with the first aspect. Economists are usually very keen of markets where prices serve the role of rationing devices. As a matter of fact, the famous first and second welfare theorems state that using a price system, together with re-distribution of wealth, is under some circumstances optimal. But if that is the case, why should we not use the price system in the health care market as well? For example, private insurers could offer several health insurance policies which are charged differently, so that people who prefer more protection can buy more expensive coverage. The argument against such a system without public insurance is not that poor people can not afford insurance. This problem might be solved by financial transfers to the poor. Instead, the main reason is what Pauly (2000) calls the 'altruistic externality', or what Breyer and Kliemt (1994) refer to as 'not being able to reject treatment'. Altruism gives rise to the following problem: Assume that a poor person is given some amount of money which he is obliged to spent on health insurance. It might be rational for this person to buy insurance which covers e.g. extensive recreation spells, beauty operations, etc. This person knows that if a serious accident occurs, he will be treated anyway. No hospital will reject him as a patient, as a consequence of the altruistic motive of society. To prevent this exploitation of altruism, the government needs to specify a catalogue of treatments which are covered by a compulsory insurance.

There is a second reason why the government should install such a basic insurance. This is the issue of risk selection. Many problems with risk selection could be solved by a well designed contract structure (see e.g. Cochrane 1995). Potentially more serious is the problem which is called 'essential adverse selection' (see e.g. van de Ven and van Vliet 1995). If consumers have better knowledge about their risks, insurers might try to attract low risks by offering cheaper policies with large deductibles, which are unattractive to high risks. This leads to under-insurance for the low risks, and thus to a welfare loss. In some cases the market may even break down. A basic compulsory insurance, which, besides, should be compulsory for all, could avoid these inefficiencies.

Thus we have good economic arguments why the government should set a catalogue of treatments in a basic insurance, while additional treatments should be covered by supplemental insurance, where prices operate as rationing devices (for a more detailed exposition, see Diamond 1992). This does not imply, however, that the basic (compulsory) insurance has to be provided by the state. It can well be done by private insurers, as long as the government assures that the poor have enough financial means to afford this insurance. Still, as the extent of coverage is determined by the government, I will speak in the following of a publicly provided basic insurance, together with complementary private insurance.

I will now turn to the question what economic theory can tell us about the limits of this basic insurance. The answer follows directly from the analysis above:

First, a basic insurance should include all those treatments which society would provide in any case, even to someone who is uninsured and who has no financial means available. A good example would be emergency treatments. I am hesitant to give more examples, because I think these should follow from a public opinion gathering process, like for example the one undertaken in Oregon (see e.g. Baur, Wang and Fitzgerald 1996). The question the public has to face is: What kind of treatment would you give to an uninsured person? Note that this is a different question from asking what kind of treatment should be included in a basic health insurance, which might well provide much more extensive treatments.

A second rationing rule follows from the effects of adverse selection, as discussed above. Economic theory shows that one way to avoid the welfare loss is that the government offers compulsory full insurance for all (Neudeck and Podczeck 1996). However, this result only holds as long as 'moral hazard' is not relevant. Moral hazard refers to the case where a patient only undergoes a particular treatment because he is insured; he would not do so if he had to pay for it himself. Then, as I have shown elsewhere (Strohmenger and Wambach 1999, 2000), such a treatment should not be included in the basic coverage, but be part of supplemental insurance. These thoughts give rise to a rule on how to decide which treatments should be included in the basic coverage, and which not. As an example, suppose that a patient has the choice between the physician on duty or the head of the medical department, who would cost some additional amount, say X. Now the patient is asked whether he would prefer to take the money X and be treated by the physician on duty, or instead receive treatment by the head of the department. If most of the patients being asked this question would prefer the money, then this is a form of treatment which should be offered via supplemental insurance. Otherwise this treatment should be included in the basic insurance. Apart from treatment by the head of medical staff, other candidates for treatments which should not be covered by basic insurance might be single room accomodation, artificial teeth or recreation stays, but also possibly excessive diagnosis, etc.

To summarize, I have outlined two questions which might guide a public process on defining rationing rules for a public insurance system: First, ask which treatments one would give to an uninsured patient without financial means, and include these into the basic coverage. Second, for any treatment (or additional treatment) find out whether most people would prefer the treatment or the money equivalent of the costs of treatment. In the latter case, this (additional) treatment should not be included in the basic coverage.

After having outlined in how far economic theory might help us in devising a health insurance system, I will now turn to the question on how I see the health insurance market, in particular the German one, evolving. For any politician, to begin a debate on rationing and rules for rationing in the health care market seems to be a non-starter. It is much easier to set budgets, reduce the size of hospitals, etc. than to explicitly discuss which treatments should not be covered for which people. On the other hand, covert or bed-side rationing with no clear rules for rationing, which is the consequence of fixed budgets, prevents the private insurance market from offering supplemental policies.[1]

Rationing will become a more and more pressing issue in the future. If the politicians will not start the public debate, then the market might do it. I expect that private insurers will take a much more active role than before by providing more extensive complementary insurance, thus indirectly defining what is not provided by the public system. This development will be similar to the pension market, where, although the government claims that pensions are secured, private insurers (and banks) have started a huge marketing campaign on private pension plans. At the same time, many new products have been introduced. It is to be expected that also private health insurers will invent new forms of supplementary policies. This in turn will lead to a redefinition of the services offered by public insurance.[2]

Many of us would probably argue that a political approach to rationing, based on democratic principles, would be the better choice. However, if politicians prefer to stick with silent rationing, it has to be someone else who brings the debate into the open. This is another way how private insurers may act complementary to the public sector.

References

Baur MN, Wang JB, Fitzgerald JF (1996) Insurance rationing versus public political rationing: The case of the Oregon Health Plan, Public Budgeting and Finance 16, pp 60–74

Besley T, Hall J, Preston I (1998) Private and public health insurance in the UK, European Economic Review 42, pp 491–497

Breyer F (1995) The political economy of rationing in social health insurance, Journal of Population Economics 8, pp 137–148

Breyer F, Kliemt H (1994) Lebensverlängernde medizinische Leistungen als Clubgüter? – Ein Beitrag zum Thema "Rationierung im Gesundheitswesen". In: Homann K (ed) Wirtschaftsethische Perspektiven I: Theorie – Ordnungsfragen – Internationale Institutionen. Duncker & Humblot, Berlin, pp 131–158

---

[1]   Under some circumstances it might be politically desired to exclude a private insurance market (see e.g. Breyer, 1995).

[2]   Such a feedback from the private on the public sector in the context of waiting lists has also been observed in England (Besley, Hall and Preston, 1998).

Cochrane JH (1995) Time-consistent health insurance, Journal of Political Economy 103, pp 445–473

Diamond PA (1992) Organizing the health insurance market, Econometrica 60, pp 1233–1254

Diamond P (1998) Symposium on the rationing of health care: 1 Rationing medical care – an economist's perspective, Economics and Philosophy 14, pp 1–26

Neudeck W, Podzceck K (1996) Adverse selection and regulation in health insurance markets, Journal of Health Economics 15, pp 387–408

Pauly MV (2000) Optimal health insurance, The Geneva Papers on Risk and Insurance 25, pp 116–127

Strohmenger R, Wambach A (1999) Gentests und ihre Auswirkungen auf Versicherungsmärkte, Zeitschrift für Wirtschafts- und Sozialwissenschaften 119, pp 121–149

Strohmenger R, Wambach A (2000) Adverse selection in the health insurance market: The role of genetic tests, Journal of Health Economics 19, pp 197–218

Ven, van de WPMM, van Vliet RCJA (1995) Consumer information surplus and adverse selection in competitive health insurance markets: An empirical study, Journal of Health Economics 14, pp 149–169

Summary Thoughts

Hartmut Kliemt

1
Withholding and Waste

We do not live in the land of plenty. Nevertheless, we sometimes waste resources as if we were living in that utopian world. However, wasting resources – in particular medical resources – is in the world of scarce resources not merely some mundane economic failure but rather a moral failure of major proportions. Inefficiency in a system of health care provision is outrageous since in our world health care (as opposed to former times) can indeed prolong life and enhance its quality. In case of waste people who would benefit from medical services are denied access to services without the necessity of denial.

It is clearly nonsensical to claim that by a more efficient allocation of resources and by eliminating all wasteful uses of resources, we could somehow "beam" ourselves into a situation where we could grant unlimited access to medical resources to all individuals. But in a state of inefficient resource allocation, we could treat additional individuals better by allocating resources more efficiently. If we intend to behave in a truly *benevolent* way to patients we are under the obligation to strive constantly for an improvement of the organization of health care provision such that all efficiency gains be realized. Benevolence presupposes efforts at efficiency.

In view of the preceding the following principle seems normatively valid:

Benevolence requires that medical care is not withheld from those who could benefit from it and who are in command of some basic entitlement to care unless all possible efficiency gains in the provision of medical care have been exploited.

2
Priorities and Withholding of Care

Once we are at the production possibility frontier in health care provision the opportunity costs of granting care to one patient consist in being unable to provide care to another patient. We must set priorities then (as discussed in Raspe, Prioritizing in Rationing, I.3). We must ask which kinds of treatments are basically more important than other forms of treatment.

It seems often quite clear how priorities should be set. For instance, emergency surgery in cases of life threatening events should in general have priority over elective forms of surgery. However, what is true more often than not need not apply always. There seem to be very important exceptions to the preceding rule of thumb. If for example a high urgency patient who needs a liver transplant is treated the opportunity cost of that treatment is typically an elective treatment forgone. It is impossible – at least for the time being – to treat a certain patient electively because the high urgency patient is preferred. Still, it is not clear at all that the priority should always be with the high urgency patient in a rational system of allocating scarce livers since survival rates between high urgency and elective patients differ much and there is no guarantee that elective patients will eventually receive a transplant.

To give but one other example, many people would think that dental care is something of lesser importance than say hip replacement in cases where the patient tends to become totally immobile. Again, even in those cases there may be special situations in which dental care might be deemed more important than hip replacement. At least the urgency of receiving certain forms of basic dental care may be very high in terms of quality of life of the patient even if the health problem might not be of a life threatening nature.

Such problems, special cases and special requirements of patients notwithstanding a rational system of resource allocation in a world of scarcity must presumably be based on priorities (or at least some mandatory standards which exactly specify what to do and what not). If we set priorities between alternative forms of *treatment* this has the advantage that we do not – possibly arbitrarily – prefer specific patients to other patients. Prioritizing certain forms of treatment over other forms of treatment all patients are – at least in a way – treated equitably. However, this advantage does not come without a certain disadvantage attached to it. The downside of the generality embodied in prioritizing forms of treatment is that we cannot always really pay attention to the specific situation of specific patients. This being said it seems still safe to say the following:

One should not withhold care without a clear and controllable scheme of priorities.

3
The five D's

Today's practice is, however, not based on setting priorities clearly and transparently. Instead of this we find the so-called big D's (as introduced in the contribution of Hunter, The Practice of Rationing Health Care in the United Kingdom, I.4). There is "deterrence" which means that the patient is scared off by unfriendly dealings. It is also often hoped that "deflection" may work, i.e. medical costs are externalized to another budget. "Dilution" or spreading the good things of medical services more thinly is operative as well. "Delay" that is installing waiting lists and letting patients wait further restricts access. Finally, the presumably most effective camouflage of "denial" by medical indication may be used, i.e. a patient who might profit from a treatment X is told that this treatment would do him more harm than good etc.

It seems that muddling through by relying on the techniques described by the five D's is possible to an astonishing extent. However, it does seem very unlikely that more serious cases of withholding care can be concealed from the views of the public by such means. That we can muddle through indefinitely seems most unlikely. We will eventually have to admit that we are withholding certain forms of care systematically.

Deterrence – unfriendly dealings – deflection – transfer to another budget – dilution – spreading treatment more thinly – delay – let the patients wait – denial of indication – just do not tell them what could be done are inferior methods of withholding care that should be avoided unless in-transparency of resource allocation is itself an aim.

4
Open vs. Concealed Withholding of Care

In the end the method of open priority setting may at least have three advantages:

First, if it is done publicly priority setting may be discussed publicly and justi-fied and criticized publicly. Second, if priorities are set publicly and discussed publicly the general public will know what to expect and what not and therefore can adapt its own plans by buying co-insurance etc. Third, the public will not be alienated from the system by the revelation that services that all should receive according to public declarations are withheld.

Quite obviously, discussing problems publicly and openly is in line with the philosophical ideals of living in an open society in which basic principles and practices are not concealed from the views of the citizens. However, in such cases like providing fundamental health care, transparency of practices might not always be regarded as a good thing. It may be deemed desirable that a certain amount of in-transparency prevails. This seems to be the case in our present systems. We tend to let physicians make decisions about who is getting what in health care. In a way, physicians are granted the legal competence to adopt the role of rationing agents of society. They allocate scarce resources in health care and weigh the interests of one patient against the interests of another one. These are doctors' decisions that do not follow from commonly known rules but must rather be made outside such rules. For otherwise the facts of scarcity and denial could not be concealed.

The question who is going to control doctors and their use or abuse of discretio-nary powers will become more pressing in the future. We must wonder whether simply conferring the power to make certain decisions on doctors is the right strategy here. If we do not think so we must presumably turn to standardization of treatment and rules that set priorities explicitly and openly. However, in that case the advantages of an in-transparent system in which doctors conceal the facts of withholding care from our views by their own discretionary decisions will be forfeited (see for related issues concerning the control of discretionary powers Baurmann, Rationing Yes, Politics No. For a Right-based Approach in Rationing Medical Goods, III.9).

The philosophical issue raised here is quite fundamental (see for related ques-tions and discussions Lübbe, Rationing – Basic Philosophical Principles and the Practice, III.10): Do we really want to know that certain people must die earlier because we have not been willing to put up sufficient resources to rescue and to treat them? Is it perhaps necessary for a society which places supreme value on the individual that the illusion of infinite solidarity with victims of brute bad luck is upheld? If that be so, the setting of priorities in public is presumably not a good idea. Moreover, standardization of treatment – desirable as it is for reasons of quality management – may have a downside in terms of enhanced transparency. In short, in an open society

transparency in the allocation of medical resources is clearly a superior strategy for unboundedly rational individuals who will deal with knowledge and facts fully rationally but not necessarily a superior strategy for boundedly rational individuals who act often emotional rather than rational.

5
Universal Coverage of What?

As long as health care is publicly provided certain principles of equal treatment that we otherwise also apply in public law may have very high standing. However, unequal treatment may be acceptable in certain cases. For instance, unequal treatment which is caused by previous decisions of those who are recipients of the treatment is much more acceptable than unequal treatment without such a justificatory basis. If by their previous behaviour individuals have somehow decided against certain measures themselves, treating them in ways that discriminate between them according to their past behavior may be deemed fair.

If people who are able to pay for their health insurance privately refuse to do so, many people would accept that they have to bear financial losses or in the more extreme cases that they might even be unable to get the treatment they need. The more consistent advocates of universal coverage would insist that even the rich or the formerly rich after losing their ability to pay for services should still receive all services necessary for securing their survival and bodily integrity. But they may nevertheless think that the rich should be held responsible for their failure to spend money on insurance.

We should be careful to note here that universal access does not necessarily mean universal coverage in terms of health insurance, though. One can well guarantee the treatment of every citizen without guaranteeing that the service will be rendered gratuitously. More specifically the state could serve as a universal guarantor of credits. Everybody who is in need of treatment – in particular in case of emergencies – would be treated. However, after being treated the state could hold the citizen financially responsible for the costs of treatment. Those who did not buy insurance against the financial risks of health care provision then would have to pay from their later earnings for the health care received before.

Suffering from severe illnesses might imply financial ruin under a scheme of universal guarantees of treatment without universal insurance. However, it cannot happen that a person for want of means would remain untreated if the person would want to be treated. Nobody would have to die because of a lack of means. True enough, those who are poor may be in debt after receiving health care services. In fact, those who are too poor to pay for health services – perhaps due to weak health – may in the last resort stay poor forever. To insure them against such financial risks of life is, however, totally different from insuring them against remaining untreated if risks for life and limb hit them. To make these distinctions is not tantamount to hold a specific position as towards which of the alternative systems of health care provision is to be preferred. It amounts, however, to a gain in clarity.

For legal-psychological reasons of stabilizing a legal order based on the notion of the overwhelming importance of the individual it may be necessary to rescue kids that fell into deep wells. For the same psychological reasons it may also be necessary to rescue grownups from such wells even though they did not buy insurance for such cases. Maybe we find out that the person who fell into the well is not able to pay for a rescue operation. Nevertheless, it seems quite unconceivable that a society like ours after checking that he is not able to pay for his own rescue would decide on letting him die.

However, it is quite well conceivable that a society like ours after rescuing a victim from an emergency situation may want to hold him responsible. In short:

The guarantee of treatment for all does not imply that all individuals must be insured. Universal coverage by insurance is not required for guaranteeing universal access to treatment.

6
Contracts and Markets

There may be market failures. Not all futures markets do exist (on the private insurance market see Fritze, Complementarity of Private and Public Insurance, IV.11, and Wambach, Rationing of Health Care and the Complementarity of Private and Public Insurance, IV.12). There are some forward contracts for which we will not find partners even though we would need them to insure risks of health care provision. A system in which the state will always serve as a guarantor of all health costs but then require reimbursement would certainly be a remedy for a lack of contracts securing future treatment. Still, markets for financial – as opposed to treatment – insurance of health risks may be missing, too.

It should be noted that some of our present structures of health care provision are not facilitating the emergence of private insurance systems. In particular global budgets with non-specified or unspecified scopes of treatment do, as Friedrich Breyer has frequently pointed out, not facilitate collateral private insurance. For, if we do not know what the state will insure us against then we do not know what to insure ourselves against on the private market. Quite clearly any of the present systems of health care provision have the perverse effect of wiping out private collateral insurance markets. They are based on maintaining officially that all patients receive the best medical care that is available at the time being. But this is a camouflage of a system of stopping at some point deemed reasonable according to the standards of doctors rather than patients. It seems obvious that

only a transparent system of withholding care in an explicit and foreseeable manner allows for a full exercise of the patients' autonomy in that it will facilitate the emergence of insurance markets for collateral treatment.